Doctors as Patients

Edited by

Petre Jones

General Practitioner
Plaistow

Foreword by
Dr Michael Shooter

Radcliffe Publishing
Oxford • Seattle

Radcliffe Publishing Ltd
18 Marcham Road
Abingdon
Oxon OX14 1AA
United Kingdom

www.radcliffe-oxford.com
Electronic catalogue and worldwide online ordering.

British Library Cataloguing in Publication Data

A catalogue record for this book is available from the British Library.

ISBN 1 85775 887 0

Typeset by Anne Joshua & Associates, Oxford
Printed and bound by TJ International Ltd, Padstow, Cornwall

Contents

Foreword   v

About the editor   vii

List of contributors   viii

Acknowledgements   x

Frontispiece
It could never happen to me
Anon   xi

Introduction
Petre Jones   xi

Part One: The Stories   1

1 Setting the scene
  Petre Jones   3

2 Personal view
  Sally Mason   7

3 Accepting who you are/learning a new identity
  Anon   9

4 Depression has many faces
  Belinda Brewer   11

5 Life can only be understood backwards
  Anon   15

6 Hope beyond . . .
  BS   19

7 Until 1996
  Rachel Vickers   21

8 My foster mother was dying
  Anon   23

9 Inside every doctor is a patient
  Joanna Watson   25

10 Running on empty
  Nikki Paiba   31

11 Since childhood
  Petre Jones   33

12 Telling the story
Anon   35

13 The other side of the sheets: a special case?
Anon   37

14 Themes from the stories
Petre Jones   39

15 Issues in treatment
Petre Jones   51

Part Two: What's It Like?   59

16 Stigma and discrimination
Lizzie Miller and Petre Jones   61

17 Easily misunderstood experiences
Petre Jones and Fiona Donnolly   67

18 Key issues for medical students and schools
Anon   73

19 Being a doctor with an illness to patients with an illness
Helen Cox, Petre Jones and Anon   85

20 GMC Health Procedures and the sick doctor
Belinda Brewer   91

21 Reflections on illness and health
Petre Jones, Joanna Watson, Helen Johnson, BS and Anon   95

Part Three: Dealing With It   103

22 Ongoing support and relapse prevention
Petre Jones, Belinda Brewer and Anon   105

23 Ideas for the dark days
Joy Pope   115

24 Flexible ways of being a GP
Petre Jones   123

25 The financial cost of illness
Declan Fox   131

26 Mental health and employment
Giselle Martinez   135

27 Doctors' Support Network
Lizzie Miller   145

28 Resources
Heike Haffmans   151

Index   191

Foreword

I had always been an up and down sort of person. On cloud nine one minute, in the depths of despair the next, for no apparent reason. I flitted from career to career, nothing seeming to fit, and wandered into medicine almost by accident. And then, in my final year of training, I wrote this poem about the distance between patient and doctor and the hopelessness of ever crossing the divide.

> What do you expect of me, or I of you?
> Will you play the part of a wife, depressed
> by a husband who drinks, a screaming child
> filing down each day to a blunt despair?
> Shall I play the part of the good doctor
> handling words like letter bombs
> mindful of the truths inside?
> We rehearse our roles in silence
> my empty cup, the ashtray, setting
> like concrete in the afternoon air.

In retrospect, I can see that the hopelessness was in me. I was on the brink of depression and needed just a push to send me over the edge. I got it. Following my consultant around the wards one night, I watched him take a dying patient in his arms and comfort him in his loneliness and his terror. 'I can't do that', I thought, 'I shall never be a doctor.' The next morning the patient asked to see me – I waited just long enough and he was dead before I got there.

I was lucky. The Dean rejected my decision to give up, told me I was depressed and sent me off for treatment. Relieved of the pressure to keep going, I dropped into a black pit that took a year out of my life and has recurred at intervals since. When it does, I am helped by a combination of medication, psychotherapy, and the care of those close to me – colleagues, friends and family. Most of all, I am helped by the opportunity they give me to talk about my illness and their ability to spot when I am heading into another depression, even before I can. That way, sometimes, I can do something about it for myself.

But others are not so fortunate. Mental illnesses are very common and doctors are just as vulnerable as anyone else. But there are fearful taboos against 'admitting' to having one (as if that were a crime). Would I ever get into medical school if I had a mental illness, would I ever get a job afterwards, would I be able to take the pressure if I did? Would patients and colleagues ever trust me? Would I ever trust myself? So doctors keep quiet about their problems and the system colludes with them, often with tragic results. No wonder that the rates of suicide in medicine are high.

We owe a great deal to the doctors who have been brave enough to tell their stories in this book, and to Petre Jones for gathering them together. Through their honesty perhaps others may feel able to share their own experiences and to seek the help of organisations like Doctors' Support Network when they need it. Is it too much to hope that the climate of the NHS itself might change, from one in which demands are made of doctors that they would not dream of making of their patients, to one in which doctors can be patients too, without fear of what it might do to their career?

The costs of this not happening are huge, but so are the benefits of allowing it to happen. Doctors do not have to be ill to know how to treat illness in others. But the doctors who can be helped with their own suffering may be more sensitive to the suffering of their patients in turn. I thought I would never be able to cradle a patient in my arms – I can now, because so many people have cradled me when I have needed it over the years.

Mike Shooter
President
Royal College of Psychiatrists
December 2004

About the editor

Petre qualified in 1985 from Sheffield University and, after house jobs, moved to East London to join the Tower Hamlets GP Vocational Training Scheme. General practice seemed a good specialty to combine with family life and Petre became a principal in 1989 and joined a successful training practice in Newham. He is a trainer and course organiser and loves teaching as much as he loves general practice. During his career he has become interested in practice management, drug abuse, mental health consultation skills and much more. He finally became diagnosed as having recurrent depression in 1998 after a suicide attempt, and moved to set up a smaller practice from scratch to improve his health. Petre now works in a two-partner training practice, but continues to teach and write occasional books, and look after himself more. He is married with five children, runs to keep fit and sometimes does lay preaching.

List of contributors

The details given in this list may appear inconsistent but each contributor was given a choice of what details they wished to appear in the book.

Belinda Brewer BSc MB BS MRCP MRCGP
General Practitioner
Chichester

Helen Cox
Trainee Psychiatrist

Fiona Donnolly
Senior House Officer, Psychiatry

Declan Fox MB MRCGP
General Practitioner
Works also in adult medicine and paediatrics

Dr Heike Haffmans
State Exam med. Germany
Flexible Trainee, Northern Deanery, UK

Dr Helen Johnson
General Practitioner

Giselle Martinez
Consultant Psychiatrist and Clinical Tutor

Sally Mason
General Practitioner

Dr Lizzie Miller AKC FRCS MRCGP BA (Psych) Dip Occ Med
Co-founder and Secretary of Doctors' Support Network

Nikki Paiba
Specialist Registrar

Joy Pope MRCGP
General Practitioner
Bolton

BS
General Practitioner

KT
General Practitioner

Rachel Vickers
Anaesthetist

Joanna Watson MA MB Bchir MFPH
Public Health Doctor

Anon

Anon

Anon
Consultant Psychiatrist

Anon
General Practitioner

Anon
General Practitioner

Anon
Medical Student

Anon
Medical Student

Anon
Trainee Physician

Anon
Trainee Psychiatrist

Acknowledgements

Special thanks to Dr Farzana Hussain for permission to use some of her material on Flexible Opportunities in General Practice. Thanks also to Dr Janet Prentis for comments on the text.

Frontispiece
It could never happen to me

Those of you who are old enough to remember the TV series 'Doctors To Be' may remember that at their medical school interviews they were shown a chart telling them that doctors have the highest rates of divorce, suicide and alcoholism. I remember watching that programme with my classmates at school during a careers talk, after I had decided to apply for medical school, and thinking – it will never happen to me, or anyone I know, because it only happens to other people.

During one of my medical school interviews I was shown that chart again, and asked how I would cope with that. I told them about how I was a well balanced individual, how my multiple interests and friends outside school made sure that things would never affect me like that. They smiled knowingly to themselves.

Now I'm only a few years out of medical school, and already amongst my peer group there have been relationship breakdowns (many), suicide, psychiatric illness (personal) and alcohol abuse.

I met a friend the other day and we could not think of a single person that we knew who were doctors and were happy. We also struggled to think of someone who was happily married.

So is this normal amongst other people of my age group who are not doctors? Did I make friends with 'the wrong crowd' at medical school? Or was becoming a doctor to blame?

Those of you who are reading this and thinking, it could never happen to me – look around you.

It probably already has.

Anon

Introduction

Petre Jones

This is a book about mental illness and some of the doctors who suffer from mental illness.

We are increasingly familiar with the issue of 'burn-out', or 'professional exhaustion' as it is better named, and its association with some of the working patterns common in the NHS. Professional exhaustion, which is a behaviour pattern rather than a mental health diagnosis, robs many of the joy of being a doctor, and deprives patients of good quality care. It is a hugely important subject, and may coexist with mental illness, but this is not a book about 'burn-out'.

What we are thinking about here is far more of a taboo subject. This book is about diagnosable, label-able mental illness such as eating disorders, affective disorders and, sometimes, psychosis. More than that, it is a book about doctors, many fully functioning practising doctors, who suffer from these illnesses, and the unique insights and problems that arise when the doctor is the patient, especially when questions of insight and judgement are blurred.

The book has come about because of the Doctors' Support Network, a self-help organisation for doctors troubled by mental illness. DSN runs support groups around the country, and runs a helpline, staffed by doctor volunteers for doctors who are needing help. We also run an email support network with a very active membership and it was on the network that we realised that as a group we have a lot of experience that we might helpfully share with the outside world. And so the vision of this book was born.

We decided to share something of our personal stories and draw out from this some of the common themes which we have encountered. We hope this will be useful to other doctors (who treat doctors and who themselves are potential patients) and students, both well and troubled, and also be of interest to health managers in the light of the current recruitment and retention problems, and in the light of DOH policy on mental health and employment. We have been truthful, honest and hopefully constructive. We have not made up examples to make a point, although some anonymisation has been done.

Some of the contributors have chosen to remain anonymous, which is fine. The stigma against mental health problems in the NHS is very strong, and of course people have a right to their own confidentiality. We are grateful that they have taken the risk of making some very personal things public. Some of the contributors have felt able to be named, and I expect everyone who reads this book to treat their decision with the respect it deserves. They are 'going public', not for personal gain (any profits from the book will go straight to Doctors' Support Network, not to any individual) or bizarre self-publicity, but in order to try to fuel a debate on the mental health of members of the medical profession, to raise awareness and possibly reduce the stigma, to the benefit of all psychiatric patients.

Here we are, a group of doctors, some working some not, who have been – and in some cases still are – mentally ill. We function well enough to write a book together and between us treat lots of patients, as well as do ordinary things like have families, go on holiday, get cross with our teenage kids. Like all psychiatric patients there is rather more to us than just our illness. We cannot be ignored as people, as doctors or as patients.

Once DSN members had contributed their personal stories and we had analysed the themes that arose from them, members of the group undertook to write chapters on detailed areas, sometimes in a traditional academic, referenced way and sometimes in a more narrative, experience-based way. We debated long and hard about this and decided that both approaches have their own validity, but because our strength as a group comes from our first-hand experience of being doctors with mental illness, the predominant style of the book should be narrative, experience-based. We also felt that poetry can express feelings that narrative text cannot, and so we have quite a generous sprinkling of poems. For me personally, creativity is greatest when I'm vulnerable or ill, and so it is that many of the poems have been written at times of major illness, and so carry an immediacy which the post hoc narrative text loses.

Some people will be drawn to this book when ill themselves and it is with them in mind that we have put a short summary at the end of each chapter. I've kept these simple and clear because I know how hard it can be to pick up a book when you have no concentration and just want to sleep.

My role as editor has been to 'hold the ring' whilst the group debated the book and its style and policies, and then guide the group through the process of creating the book. I have left the personal stories almost completely unchanged, written a couple of themed chapters myself, and added the chapter summaries. My aim has been to let the voices of the contributors speak for themselves. This has led to what we always knew would be a rather anarchic, unconventional book, but that's what the group are like. Radcliffe have worked hard to knock us into readable shape.

All the authors have written to the best of their knowledge and research, but we are only human, so please don't sue us if something goes wrong for you after reading our thoughts. Neither are we lawyers, so if you need to speak to one, speak to a lawyer, not us.

This is not an easy book to read. It was not an easy book to write. Some of the stories are sad, some will make you angry, and some are simply hard to believe. We hope you will feel that some of your assumptions are challenged, and we hope that some will be moved to act. Above all, I hope that readers will learn that mental illness need be no more of a taboo than a broken leg, and that even we, as strong clever resourceful professionals, are heir to human frailty and illness, like anyone else. Patients can be doctors: doctors are patients.

Summary

- This book is about mental illness in doctors and arose from the Doctors' Support Network, a group of doctors troubled by mental illness.
- The authors are sharing personal stuff for the benefit of the profession as a whole, and we should respect their stories and their gift.
- Sometimes the book is objective, and sometimes it is about personal narratives. Both approaches help us understand the issues.
- Poetry is used to express things that other forms cannot.
- This is not an easy book to read, or to write, but we hope it reinforces our shared humanity.

Further information relating to this book is available at www.radcliffe-oxford/doctorsaspatients

Petre Jones
December 2004

Part One

The Stories

Chapter 1

Setting the scene

Petre Jones

Mental illness is difficult to understand unless you have close experience of it, and to understand it in the familiar context of members of the medical profession is even harder unless you have been involved in such a situation. Doctors are traditionally strong and almost by definition have achieved a high degree of 'success' by most standards. How is it that doctors can fall prey to mental illness? How are we to comprehend the nature of this intrusion into our comfortable world? The personal stories contained in this book give a clear insight into the coming of illness into the world of ordinary individuals. This chapter will try to give a broader perspective, into which those individuals fit.

A study by Caplan in 1994[1] looked at stress levels in GPs, consultants and health service managers. They found that 47% of the study population reported high levels of stress on the general household questionnaire, with 29% suffering 'clinically significant' levels of stress. Of the consultants and GPs, 27% scored >8 on a hospital anxiety and depression scale (1–7 normal, 8–10 mild, 11–14 moderate, 15–21 severe anxiety/depression) and, worryingly, 14% of GPs and 5% of consultants displayed suicidal thinking. Women report more mental illness than men, but overall an estimated 25% of doctors are vulnerable to mental health problems.

The numbers trip off the tongue, but consider a fairly typical teaching hospital with, say, 175 consultants, in a typical district with 125 GPs. That works out as 75 'vulnerable' professionals on the edge of formal mental illness, or 27 professionals having suicidal ideation, in one health district at any one time. That is quite a problem.

But how does this compare with the rest of the population? We are all heir to the frailties of human flesh after all. Murray[2] looked at admission rates for mental illness for doctors, and compared them to a control group of non-medical professionals. The study found admission rates were twice as high for the doctors, and, revealingly, that the doctors were more likely to be admitted via self-referral or by non-GP referral.

A similar story is told by relative risks of suicide, as shown in Table 1.1,[3] derived from a meta-analysis of suicide studies.

Table 1.1 **Relative risks of suicide in doctors**

Rates compared with the general population	Male doctors	1.1–3.4
	Female doctors	2.7–5 .7
Rates compared to other professionals	Male doctors	1.5–3.8
	Female doctors	3.7–4.5

Why should this vulnerability be so great when, after all, doctors are intelligent resourceful people who have jumped over many hurdles just to get to be doctors? Bellini and colleagues[4] in the US looked at psychological indicators in people starting internship posts. He found that initial enthusiasm gave way to feelings of depression, anger and fatigue after only five months in post, despite the cohort starting the jobs with better than average scores. This not unsurprising finding is influenced by professional culture factors, job factors and personal factors.

The job we do is inherently stressful. The work is intense and people's lives and wellbeing depend on our actions and the choices we make. The importance of the work tends to lead to a sense of being responsible, adding to stress and a tendency to work longer than contracted hours. Our work also brings us up against critical life events for others such as deaths, disability and emotional distress on a daily basis whatever our specialty, and traditionally we have only rudimentary ways of dealing with the inner effects of this on us.

Organisational issues within medicine compound this. Frequent job changes in trainees compound lack of support and increase their stress[5] and substantial and persistent organisational and technological change across the service is bad for everyone. 'The management of change is an art that the NHS has yet to perfect.'[6]

The culture of medicine compounds rather than alleviates the damaging effects of these stressors. After a major incident it is rare for a medical team to debrief and support its members. The work keeps coming, time is at a premium and we just don't see the need. In my role as course organiser of a GP training scheme I help run case discussion groups looking at the emotional baggage left behind for junior doctors in both hospital and GP settings after such events. Suicides and deaths and unsupportive attitudes of colleagues are the most frequent causes of problems, which are often only reported weeks or even months after the index event. Difficult emotions are stored up and ruminated upon. Almost never is a major incident within a department discussed in a supportive team setting, exploring emotions raised and looking for actions to take. Usually the doctor, and other staff, just dust themselves off, over a coffee if they're lucky, and throw themselves into the next challenge. This may be okay for some personality types, but for the vulnerable 25% at least, it is storing up trouble. This silent stoicism happens in all specialties as well as in general practice, where even apparently close partnerships can be remarkably closed to emotional discussion. A medical culture of needing to be 'manly and tough' and minimising one's own symptoms, whilst feeling that patients overestimate their symptoms, seems to be learned in medical school.[6] One general exception to this 'don't talk about it' rule seems to be the one-to-one relationship between GP registrar and trainer, where talking and even an informal psychotherapeutic relationship can happen.

Competition and rivalry between colleagues makes mutual support harder. In the training grades we compete with each other to pass exams, which are themselves often peer-referenced, where you are competing against each other for a set proportion of passes. We compete with each other for the 'best' jobs. This is not conducive to mutual support. In senior grades and in GP partnerships we compete in departmental politics and encounter those interpersonal difficulties that can make working life so difficult.

And then there's stigma, and prejudice. Of course no one would admit to being prejudiced against mental illness, but stigma in the medical profession was considered so grave that in a report on the tragic suicide of one doctor with mental health problems it was considered a major contributory cause.[7] Other chapters in this book look at this issue in more detail, but suffice to say that if a doctor feels they would be stigmatised by disclosure of personal distress they are not likely to seek support, which is exactly what happens.[8]

Not all doctors succumb to mental illness, so what is it about those who do that makes them vulnerable? Choice of career at an early age is associated with vulnerability, and many authors have postulated psychological scenarios, arising in childhood experience, which can not only underlie career choice but also make someone more susceptible to the effects of the stresses of the work.

A medical career may serve as a defence against feelings of anxiety or impotence resulting from the experience of illness or death in family members.[9,10]

Bowlby[11] described 'compulsive care giving', in which the doctor, having experienced unsatisfactory parental attachments, gives care to others that they themselves never received as a child, and Malan[12] talks of the 'helping profession syndrome' in which other people's needs are seen as demands which they have to satisfy. If they are unable to satisfy those needs of others they experience a sense of failure and become liable to depression. The idea that we as professionals have to make it all better for everyone else is quite familiar, and works if we can confidently improve the lives of our patients. If we cannot, we have failed.

One can go on speculating about personal traits which lead people to become health professionals, but the point is simple enough: that medicine for many of us is a type of compensation for, or occupational therapy for, psychological scars. Of course, we all have our neurotic traits, that is part of what it means to be human, it is just that for some of us those traits interact with our working lives to the extent that as a profession we suffer from a heavy excess of psychological morbidity, including suicides.

A different perspective can be seen in an Old Testament story. Seven centuries BC, one of history's great empire builders, Nebuchadnezzar, King of Babylon, built an empire from the Indus valley to the Nile. Biblical and archaeological evidence stands testimony to his conquests and building triumphs. However, later in his reign it seems he became ill. He left his palace and lived rough, neglecting his self-care, letting his nails and hair grow. He was clearly unable to govern, and remained in this state for a period of 'seven times', however long that may be. Eventually he returned to a state of mental health, and his officials went to find him. He was restored to the throne and, as one would expect from a story in an ancient document, he became even more successful as a ruler after his illness. The point of retelling this story is simple. Whatever the causes of the excessive psychiatric morbidity in medical professionals, the majority of illnesses from which we suffer – affective disorders, addictions, eating disorders – if treated, leave the patient with a reasonably preserved level of social functioning. The King of Babylon did well with his illness. He was allowed to recover and was eventually restored to his former role. So too with doctors suffering from mental illness; with proper treatment, we stand a good chance of being restored to work. It is helpful if those around us can allow us to get on with it and await our recovery without adding stigma to our burden.

References

1 Caplan RP (1994) Stress, anxiety, and depression in hospital consultants, general practitioners, and senior health service managers. *BMJ.* **309**: 1261–3.

2 Murray RM (1977) Psychiatric illness in male doctors and controls. Admission rates for mental illness in doctors. *British Journal of Psychiatry.* **131**: 1–10.

3 Lindeman S *et al.* (1996) A systematic review on gender-specific suicide mortality in medical doctors. *British Journal of Psychiatry.* **168**: 274–9.

4 Bellini LM *et al.* (2002) Variation in mood and empathy during internship. *JAMA.* **287**: 3143–6.

5 Firth-Cozens J *et al.* The effect of 1-year rotations on stress in preregistration house officers. *Hosp Medicine.* **62**(5): 305.

6 Donaldson LJ (1994) Sick doctors (editorial). *BMJ.* **309**: 557–8.

7 North East London Strategic Health Authority (2003) *Report of an independent inquiry into the care and treatment of Daksha Emson and her daughter Freya.* www.nelondon.nhs.uk/documents/de_inquiry_report.pdf

8 Court C (1994) British study highlights stigma of sick doctors. *BMJ.* **309**: 561–2.

9 Pfeffer CR (1983) Early adult development in the medical student. *Mayo Clinic Proceedings.* **58**: 127–34.

10 Gabbard GO (1985) The role of compulsiveness in the normal physician. *JAMA.* **254**: 2926–9.

11 Bowlby J (1977) The making and breaking of affectionate bonds. *British Journal of Psychiatry.* **130**: 201–10.

12 Malan DH (1995) *Individual Psychotherapy and the Science of Psychodynamics.* Butterworth, London.

Summary

- Mental illness is common amongst doctors, with about 25% vulnerable to it.
- Suicide rates are between 2 and 4 times those of other professionals.
- The work of medicine is inherently stressful.
- The culture of medicine is not generally supportive.
- Stigma and prejudice exacerbate mental ill-health.
- Personality traits in some doctors make them more vulnerable.
- Most ill doctors either make a reasonable recovery or reach a functioning chronic or recurrent state.

Chapter 2

Personal view

Sally Mason

Why do idealistic, intelligent, resourceful young adults choose a career which cares for their physical and emotional wellbeing so badly? Youth never fears for death, but doctors have a high risk of occupational misery with long hours, outmoded practices, stiff upper lip and vast numbers of sick people at their medical mercy every day!

When you start out in medicine, you work according to the book, but gradually the gifts of intuition and expertise develop. The demands of family, government and patients take more and more from us all. Often there is not even the time or energy to continue those hobbies and activities which previously 'defined' you as an individual. Some burn out – switch off and withdraw from partners and patients except for the absolutely necessary or find solace in information technology. Others care too much and turn the emotion back on themselves, leading inevitably to depression. The innate sensitivity and desire to care, followed by exposure to so much suffering – in the world, your domain and your family – adds up to a haemorrhage of 'brain juice'. It is silly to think that one has to have been ill to better empathise with a patient, but having had 'depression' one can sense it in others' eyes, and care and comfort – if not cure. The wounded healer can be a better healer, but s/he needs to be respected. In the same way other gifts are admired – ability to understand an ECG, the renal tubule, chemotherapy – why are the emotional and spiritual not? You could say that such should be the remit of the priest or counsellor – but so can the ECG and the renal tubule be the domain of the technician or scientist. Having both a medical training and other gifts is valid and powerful.

Some of us will find the intuitive side of medicine second nature after a while, and empathy is a useful tool. What comes first? The ability to recognise suffering in one's fellows, or a tendency to melancholia, being overwhelmed by the misery of the human condition? Does one necessarily beget the other and vice versa? When caring, empathic doctors find they get overloaded with emotions, who is there to put the mess back in proportion? Patients 'vomit' their problems and symptoms all over us, and we have to clear it up. We can help them see how to clear up the next lot themselves, but we've already got some in our laps.

So, I therefore ask, where is the Occupational Health Department for General Practice? Are we not at least as vulnerable as our white coat colleagues? Where is the supervision that psychotherapists have? Where do we put all the pain, anger and suffering at the end of the day but inside ourselves? Some doctors who crack under the strain do not ask for help, or realise that help is possible. It is not easy for us to ask colleagues for help, and admit fragility, nor is it easy to realise what is happening. The fear overlying the sick doctor is immense, shown by reactions from 'well' colleagues as well as our reactions to ourselves, and should be exposed and excised. The waste in individual potential, talent and aspiration is immense and the loss to the nation a scandal.

How about a new code for the millennium? Trust, self-awareness, admittance of weakness to others in confidence, and compassion shown to colleagues will change the climate. Put you, yourself at the top of the needs pile, not family, government, patients, the forces that drive us, and we will maintain a physically and mentally competent, caring medical workforce we can all want to be part of.

6 July 1998

Chapter 3

Accepting who you are/learning a new identity

Anon

I am a consultant psychiatrist, married to a GP, with two kids in primary school.

I have experienced recurrent depressions since my teens. Apart from having to restart a year in medical school after one bout, these were not bad enough to keep me from work till 10 years ago.

Around my late twenties I had bouts when I was unable to concentrate on anything, slept poorly, was irritable and tearful and was totally lacking in confidence and self-esteem. On the worse days I felt physically ill, aching all over, my eyesight seemed blurred, my throat hurt. I blamed all these symptoms on pressure of work, being unsuited to the job or premenstrual syndrome (despite little objective relationship to my actual cycle). I neglected my appearance and stopped enjoying my food, although I ate vast amounts of chocolates and cakes. I tried evening primrose oil, B6, etc. People started noticing I was not myself.

Despite having my MRCPsych and spending lots of time explaining depression to patients and relatives I was totally unable to recognise it in myself, and it was almost a shock when a friend suggested I saw a GP, who agreed and suggested I take antidepressants. Still I did not expect them to work. I decided instead to leave higher training and work as a staff grade, convinced I was inadequate as a person and almost incompetent as a doctor, despite extensive evidence to the contrary.

I remember vividly a moment on a holiday in the Italian Lakes which should have been wonderful. I was with a good man who loved me, career going well, the sun was shining, the scenery glorious, good food and nothing to worry about. Except I was unable to enjoy it. I had a feeling of numbness and emptiness. I stood gazing over Lake Como with tears streaming down my face and thinking if this is what life is like I don't want to go on living. That frightened me so much I saw privately a psychiatrist I respected, who again suggested antidepressants. It also frightens me in retrospect that I told no one of my suicidal feelings until the psychiatrist asked and was able to function almost normally (almost on automatic pilot) at work despite this despair.

After a few months on antidepressants I suddenly realised I had been fairly miserable on and off for a long time and had variously explained it on pressure of work, exams, bereavement – anything really. I started believing in myself again and re-entered higher training, obtaining my CCST without difficulty and with excellent references. I even had time to do an MBA with the Open University – as well as having two children. I had a further bout of depression after the birth of my daughter when I delayed restarting antidepressants because I wanted to breast-feed. I did not make the same mistake twice and after my second pregnancy I took antidepressants prophylactically when my son was born.

I was well on antidepressants for approximately five years despite lots of life events. My confidence soared and I became very involved in medical politics and academic activities. I saw myself as at least equal to the best of my peers. Unfortunately, over the last five years I have had two more big bouts of depression and this summer a rather strange experience which was probably what the textbooks call a mixed affective state. I am currently on two different antidepressants and sodium valproate (as a mood stabiliser) and seeing a psychologist.

I am also trying to reorganise my life so that further swings will not cause so much disruption, and to increase my exposure to work I find stimulating while decreasing the kind of work I find most harmfully stressful (most of my community clinical work). I now see a psychiatrist at a different hospital fairly regularly which helps since my GP felt a little overwhelmed and I felt I was almost treating myself before. I am finding it hard to come to terms with the fact that the work I think I am pretty good at might be contributing to my relapses and suffering a sense of loss when I think of all I am giving up. Maybe will go back one day . . .

At present I feel I am not sure who I am. It seems obvious that five years ago I became a consultant and perhaps my personality and bipolar genes (there is a family history) make me unsuited to the pressures of being a community psychiatrist. I am trying hard not to feel I am a failure. On my better days (thankfully more often now) I can recognise that I have not failed as a person and I am not totally inadequate. In other areas of my life I can take pressure that would make others crumble and it is specific stresses that I need to avoid. Sometimes I find myself thinking, perhaps with the right combination of drugs I will be OK and able to manage – but I know that is not realistic. I am also trying to train myself to take more exercise and eat more sensibly. It may seem trivial to some, but the drugs can make you put on weight, and when your self-esteem is low this is not exactly helpful and can almost counteract their beneficial effects.

I am very lucky that my husband, GP and work colleagues have been so supportive, insightful and understanding. I know many others in my position cannot reorganise their lives in such a way that they continue to cope with stimulating yet stressful activities that are right for them while discarding the harmful stresses. Too many doctors find the system so inflexible that they have to leave medicine altogether. This is a sad loss for the individuals, the profession and society. However, there are others who will find that they are not suited to medicine at all and it will be a challenge for them to recognise that this is not the end and they are not failures, just not doctors. There are many facets to a human life and every diamond is different.

There is very little practical help available for doctors with particular needs, and even less informed careers counselling. This is one of the things that I hope our campaigning can change. The UK departments of health have in theory embraced the concept of promoting diversity and flexibility in the way we work. We will soon see if they mean it.

Chapter 4

Depression has many faces

Belinda Brewer

Depression has many faces. It makes some people very angry or irritable. It makes other people very flat or numb. There's also the classical form of being very sad and tearful. I'm a mixture of everything. It's like being caught in a fishing net and the more you fight, the more entangled you become. Severe depression robs you of life and the ability to give or receive. I knew that my late twenties were literally disappearing and there was nothing I could do to be part of them.

I'm 34 now. I guess my ambition to be a doctor dates back to when I was nine or ten. I wanted to be a doctor, I wanted to help people. I love contact with people and I suppose it was this cliched view that motivated me to apply to medical school. Academically I probably peaked around 27 when I took the MRCP postgraduate exam. Following this I had a huge career decision to make. Was I to continue in the highly competitive world of general hospital medicine and cardiology, sacrificing any chance of a normal life that balances work and pleasure?

It was around this time that I started losing weight. I was having early morning sweats, I wasn't sleeping, I was always anxious. I thought maybe I had some kind of cancer.

It was while sitting in a lecture on depression that it suddenly occurred to me that the lecturer was describing me: 'That's what is happening to me'. I came out of the lecture terrified. A friend rang the psychiatrist giving the lecture and arranged an appointment for that same afternoon. It did not take long for her to confirm that I was suffering from a depressive episode. She recommended I start taking a course of antidepressants. I did not even have a GP at the time. I kept it a secret for a year, I felt so ashamed.

It got to the point where I couldn't even open the door to visitors. I was unable to manage a full day's work. I'd do an hour and come home, then go back. I couldn't open the mail, I was living a nightmare.

Mental illness was always a taboo subject in my family. When I became ill I questioned my grandmother and found out there was a significant family illness of depression and mental health problems on my father's side. On my mother's side there were also problems relating to alcohol and possibly depression. I felt there were huge expectations around my future career and here I was, completely unable to make simple daily decisions like whether to make a cup of tea. Other than my work I had little other structure and interests. I had lost touch with many friends, I no longer played any of the sports that had been such a large part of my life up until I qualified.

I'd taken all my exams and still loved being a doctor, but I was unable to continue with my potentially high-flying career.

I remember thinking, 'Help, I'm just reacting to life. I am not an active participant.'

One course of antidepressants just didn't resolve the problem. In retrospect, I should've been signed off sick, but I wasn't. Things just continued to deteriorate, and 15 months after that first lecture I took an overdose of over-the-counter tablets. It was a scream for help, because I had the knowledge to kill myself properly, but I didn't.

Following the overdose I was admitted to the hospital I was working in. That was one of the all-time low points. The consultant I had worked for was covering that night, he came in and I remember him crying, the staff had no idea I was so depressed. I went back to work eight days later and within an hour of arriving I was huddled in the corner of a dark room.

I was eventually referred to a psychiatrist who admitted me to a private acute psychiatric hospital. That was so frightening.

I lasted four days and discharged myself. Over the course of the next two years, there were antidepressants, psychiatrists and numerous crisis admissions, but I just didn't get any better. I made some very serious suicide attempts during that time, including self-injecting powerful drugs, and even attempted hanging myself.

I was put on lots of high dose antidepressants that, when taken away, precipitated severe depression. As a consequence of the antidepressants, I can become quite 'high'. I have to watch out for the signs of this elation, as in addition to feeling very happy I get very hyped up, excitable, I spend lots of money, I'm irritable and I tease people.

So I have to find a balance between the highs and lows. Last August I became very depressed and agitated. I was very sick and vividly suicidal. I needed to be admitted to hospital but the funding for admission to the hospital where my psychiatrist worked had been taken away. I became more distressed at the thought of admission to an unknown hospital an hour's drive from my home and friends. I was convinced at the time that dying was a better option. My GP and psychiatrist thought leaving me at home was the lesser of the risks. Unfortunately I took a morphine overdose.

Following this episode I decided to look for a new consultant who could provide a more comprehensive package. I knew if the situation did not change I would be dead. I started my desperate search. I knew I needed an NHS consultant who could admit me when necessary, outside of the area I worked, somewhere I could be treated as a normal patient, not a doctor.

I eventually found a hospital that was a commutable distance but in a different health authority to the one I worked in. The new consultant psychiatrist is female, really supportive and very dynamic. I have a very committed GP who has been an enormous source of strength. She has consistently given wise advice and guidance. My health and quality of life has improved immensely with their help. It is essential to find a GP and psychiatrist you trust if you suffer from a chronic mental health problem.

Over the last seven years I've changed jobs five times. I went from being a physician, to an A&E registrar, to a palliative care job and finally to general practice.I have worked full-time and then changed to part-time and I have tried to find a balance between the job I love, my illness and my sporting hobbies.

Many of the people I have worked with start off being supportive but when I need time off the support often wanes. As a flexible trainee in the hospital I have found you are treated as a second-class citizen. There is the attitude 'I wish I could have time off if I get stressed'. There is little appreciation that depression is not just feeling a little stressed. You cannot concentrate, remember things, make decisions or find any part of the day enjoyable.

I have now retrained as a GP and work part-time. General practice has been more supportive and understanding of my difficulties. The balance I have now seems to be working well, I work between two and a half and three and a half days per week as a salaried GP in a local practice. I also do one clinic session in a cardiology clinic; this keeps up my interest in my favourite area of medicine.

Patients have never been at risk and the one thing I've always been good at is my job. We're losing doctors and it's so damaging to the profession. We're losing doctors that are sick, we're losing doctors that are burnt out, they are retiring earlier or just not going into the profession after medical school.

Doctors have a tremendous fear of mental health. There is the fear of peer criticism and the belief that doctors don't get ill. At medical school you're pushed and pushed academically, but you don't mature emotionally.

I absolutely love being a doctor. Listening to people and not judging them. Being a doctor and not being able to work robs you of more than just your health.

This is not just a job, being a doctor is fundamentally integrated into everything we are.

Chapter 5

Life can only be understood backwards

Anon

Life can only be understood backwards, but it must be lived forwards

Kirkegaard

In *Tales of the Dervishes* by Idries Shah there is a story called Fatima the Spinner and the Tent. Fatima has all sorts of adverse experiences in her life, repeatedly starting afresh and gaining new skills; at the end, she is set a task which uses all her skills and brings a happy ending.

I'm still waiting for the happy ending. Don't get me wrong. I am doing quite well. I'm able to work full-time, I have a good salary, creature comforts, a wife who loves me. Every so often I remember that having enough to eat and drink makes me better off than huge numbers of human beings.

I lack confidence and self-esteem and my mood goes down at times. I've found alcohol can be a quick fix but causes problems of its own. My problems are not neat and circumscribed. Slowly I have found some ways to erode them or bypass them; I am still learning.

When I was having a gloomy time leading up to my A levels, I thought that this low feeling was the worst possible thing. I developed the idea that becoming a psychiatrist would help people having these low feelings, which would be a 'good thing' to do. I had just started seeing a psychiatrist myself, who clearly did not think much of my plan, but kindly did not try to dissuade me. I didn't know anything about medicine (or psychiatry) but went ahead with my career. Of course there have been pitfalls, particularly overidentification with the patient and predicating my self-esteem on making patients feel better, but I think I have avoided major excess and certainly prefer to err in that direction than display callous indifference, disdain or simple boredom.

I was not prepared for the fact that my first wife would become mentally ill herself, and that she could not accept that she had a mental illness. I blamed myself for making her ill and felt rejected by her rejection of a diagnosis and attention from my chosen profession. I decided that it would be better for both of us to get divorced. This precipitated my most severe spell of depression ending in inpatient care and ECT. The recovery room had an outside window and I remember waking up and noticing that the sky was blue – everything had been monochrome before, dark grey shading into black.

Although I got better, my life took a wrong turn. While in hospital I was visited by a woman who began coming on to me and a relationship started when I was in a very vulnerable state. She was the psychiatrist who had treated me before admission. This ultimately did not work out and led to another 'failure'.

I managed to get a consultant level post, but this was a bad move. Things I had been told about the job did not match how it really was. The relationship started in hospital finally foundered. I felt lost and floundering. I was drinking too much and this was apparent to my colleagues. I went through various attempts to make my job workable without success and I was asked to leave with a lump sum – paid off. I negotiated that I would use the same money as salary and do some non-clinical work while I looked for another job. I did manage to get a non-clinical post, and got through the health screening. I immediately ran into the further problems with lack of supervision and lack of clarity about my role. I found out that my boss was notorious for being difficult and after a good three-month probationary report and ten days after buying a flat, at six months I was told that I would not be taken on permanently. I decided to go back to clinical work, sat in on some local ward rounds, and got a locum consultant job.

I had great difficulty getting a substantive job until I changed one of my referees. My goal was to stick it for a minimum of three years. I stuck my first post for four years, then made an internal move and stayed another few years. My clinical career was starting to come together.

I had seen a few psychiatrists, who did their best but had difficulty coping with me because I didn't just have classical depressive episodes with complete recovery inbetween like the textbooks say (and what they are trained to deal with). I often had low-grade 'neurotic' (i.e. unimportant, easily ignored) symptoms, and drinking as well. I ended up seeing a professor who was expert in treatment-resistant depression, even though he was a long way from where I lived. I saw him briefly and infrequently, but he was very helpful. I saw a substance misuse consultant for a while. I got referred for cognitive therapy, which was great. I expected something very white coat and dispassionate, and was not prepared for how emotional and draining it was. It was the right therapy at the right time, and I had an excellent therapist. I started writing poetry regularly and going to poetry workshops. After the cognitive therapy ended, I went to a private therapist trained in psychosynthesis who used guided imagery/visualisation, which I think is very powerful, and who encouraged me to use art materials in sessions. She was affirming, looking at strengths, and honest. That ended when I moved away to my current job.

After a succession of failed relationships, I now have a wife who loves me and supports me. I have built up my non-work life, although there is room for further work there. I have moved into a type of work where I can spend longer time with fewer patients, which suits me better. My alcohol consumption has decreased significantly. I know I'm never going to be happy or even content much of the time, but every day I make a note of some instances of mastery and of pleasure (it is rare I can't find at least one example of each). I managed to get off all medication at one point; currently I am on one of the newer antidepressants with few side effects, and am not in a hurry to come off it. I think that things can and will improve.

What I have learned

- It's your life, it's up to you to get it right.
- Other people can help.
- If the help isn't helping, change the help.
- Creativity (writing, art, music) and spirituality/faith are powerful allies.
- Timing and sequencing are important.
- Unpicking vicious cycles and constructing virtuous cycles can be a very slow process; keep at it.

Things to do

- Go on an assertiveness training course (books are unlikely to help).
- Find professionals who help.
- Do things you enjoy (as long as they don't harm others).
- Do things you are good at (as long as they don't harm others).
- Avoid people who make you feel bad.

Chapter 6

Hope beyond . . .

BS

Writing this I realise I've had a mental illness for five years. It is only recently that I have come to feel I am a person first with mental health problems in addition. I became depressed while working as a half-time principal in general practice when a number of factors came together and, as well as great irritability at home, I began to struggle with work demands. For a while I gave myself permission to be miserable. Despite trying very hard to renegotiate hours it seemed that the only solution was to resign and think again.

My own GP, a gentle soul, gave me the fluoxetine I asked for, but did not realise how deep my despair was. Intervention by a work colleague meant I saw a consultant who visited me at home. A CPN became involved but somehow the various drugs and support did not lift my mood as hoped. I slogged on, trying to work my six months' notice but just didn't make it, and six weeks before the date I was due to finish I was admitted to a private clinic away from my practice area.

As far as this period is concerned, my mind is fairly blank. I was apparently becoming catatonic, had ECT, felt well enough in a short while to bring myself home only to be readmitted a while later. I did not really get on with the very authoritarian consultant and I have a feeling we were mutually glad to part ways.

The new millennium saw me trying to function and returning to a different practice as a 2–3 session retainer. I had got fairly good at hiding my deep despair and at the end of that year people knew I was struggling but no one saw the suicide attempt coming. I had many different tablets by now. I had it all planned, notes read. I saw the consultant on Friday. He did not ask about suicidal thoughts so I didn't tell him. Instead I set up the certainty of an undisturbed day and swallowed a cocktail of about 100 tablets. Five days ventilated in ITU, dialysed and resuscitated, meant I woke up to life – I was not happy. When physically well enough I was transferred to a Priory hospital where I spent the best part of the next eight months.

More drug changes, very comfortable surroundings, an extensive therapy programme; all helped, as well as forays into EMDR and NLP, but I seemed to need all this help just to clamber back to coping mode. On discharge I coped, I was with my husband and three children who had to reclaim the function of this Mummy person.

Again the Autumn approached and my mood struggled, and a new NHS consultant (the previous one had retired) became involved, talking of admission under the MHA if necessary. I avoided the section but not the hospital stay. Four months in an NHS psychiatric unit got my medication to the best it had been and the limited resources were stretched by committed staff to provide a reasonable service. I was discharged rather battle-worn and weary.

It has been a long, slow process of rehabilitation. I am exceedingly lucky to have a brilliant psychologist whom I still see two times a week. I am encouraged by his statement that the recurrence rate in those who have CBT after a severe depression falls to 18%. (I almost daren't write that it's an 80% recurrence rate for those with no CBT.)

It took 15 months from discharge for me to pluck up the courage to work again – in a very limited way, as a returner to general practice. I've recently coped with a number of life events without falling apart.

I want to believe for all of us there's hope.

Chapter 7

Until 1996

Rachel Vickers

Until 1996 my knowledge of mental illness was limited to doing psychiatry as a medical student, giving anaesthetics for ECT and observing illness in friends and relations. The most valuable things I now realise are that no one can really understand what it is like to be depressed unless they have been, that it can happen to anyone, and that everyone's story is different.

Until May 1996 my life had run a fairly 'normal' course. Following graduation I pursued a career in anaesthetics and had progressed well. I was a senior registrar, had been married for eight years and gave birth in May 1996 to my first (planned) child. My pregnancy had been straightforward although I stopped working at 23 weeks because of tiredness and sickness. I had an emergency Caesarian section for foetal distress. None of this was a particular emotional problem for me but by eight weeks postnatally I had a developed postnatal depression, which developed into a very severe and protracted illness. I did not eat or speak for days at a time and was frequently suicidal. I was admitted to the coronary care unit following an overdose of lithium. Unfortunately the depression did not appear to respond to any treatment – tricyclics, SSRIs, lithium, or ECT. It was unusual in being cyclical which made it difficult to manage as I would seem to be getting better but then deteriorate again. I was in hospital for nearly 18 months in a mother and baby unit, but once recovery started I became well quickly and have not suffered from depression since, including following the birth of my second child in 2000.

I believe that some doctors do have specific problems if they develop a mental illness but this wasn't the case for me. I had a GP who had no difficulty (at least from my perspective) in dealing with a fellow doctor and was caring throughout (not that we always agreed with each other). Retrospectively I realise how much I could trust him, particularly when it came to the difficult decision about having another baby and the anxiety through my second pregnancy and postpartum period. He agreed during my second pregnancy that it was inappropriate for me to see a psychiatrist in the Trust I was working for. The anaesthetist overseeing my training was also helpful – it was he who ensured I was paid sick leave when I was unable to return to work following maternity leave and also returned to work very gradually and was totally supervised as I did so. Having met other doctors who have suffered from mental illness and following news from DSN I realise I may have been lucky and wonder whether the reason I now hold the consultant post of my choice reflects this.

I have come into contact with many non-medical people suffering mental illness, both whilst I was ill and subsequently during my involvement with the local MIND group, both as a user and, now, trainer. Whilst I agree that doctors have particular problems when they are mentally ill, I think it is important to realise that non-medical people also have poor management. Most mothers do not get admitted to a mother and baby unit. I was spared the weekly interrogation session (sorry, ward round) because of my status.

In conclusion then, yes, doctors may have specific problems which may be poorly dealt with. However, in my case it just needed a good caring GP, an admission to a mother and baby unit, and help from work to overcome these problems. And let us not forget the 'average' mental illness patient, who also gets a raw deal.

Chapter 8

My foster mother was dying

Anon

Back in 1999. She was my last link to some of the best bits of my past and I knew I wouldn't be able to hack it. Her reluctance to accept help from anyone else coupled with a determination to die at home made my life impossible. My daytime job was as a palliative care SHO at the local hospice, a mixed blessing, as others could relate to what I was going through but at the same time I saw examples of care that were so much better than my single-handed attempts. So, in preparation for the inevitable bereavement I asked for help. I thought it was the sensible thing to do, acknowledging the role this woman had played in a traumatic childhood and recognising the depths of despair and loneliness that her death was likely to provoke. That was a decision I have regretted many times until recently when, finally, four years on, I am beginning to find peace.

It started off OK, seeing a liaison psychiatrist as I had many somatising symptoms. I found it hard to trust him but after nearly a year felt we were starting to make progress. I last saw him in November when he said he would see me again before Christmas. The next I heard was a letter through the post saying that he had referred my case to the GMC.

By this time I was a GP registrar and my trainer was amazing. He never once doubted me and my own GP was also supportive. So I waited, and waited . . . Eventually in March I gave up and phoned the MPS . . . two weeks later I got a letter from the GMC's solicitors, all in legal speak, which basically said that there were concerns about my practice and I had to agree to two assessments. I was also encouraged to send in evidence supporting my case, which I did.

The first assessment was in London, by a retired psychiatrist who had worked with my trainer's brother. A warm, Christian man, he politely invited me to see him, giving alternative options if I couldn't make the proposed date. He sat and listened to me calmly and patiently for 90 minutes as I poured out my grief (my foster mother having by now died) and my anger at the way the system had treated me. We parted on good terms.

The second assessment was on my birthday! What a present. This time there was no choice and I was summoned to Birmingham on two consecutive days despite my protests at the distance. The first day I underwent various psychometric tests and the second day I had the actual assessment. This took the form of three and a half hours of cross-examination about dates and events of the past, things that I had long since tried to suppress. It concluded with her stating that she probably needed further info but that the report would be written within six weeks.

There then followed a long period of silence apart from an unreasonable request from the second assessor to have access to my school reports and other info that I declined on the grounds of invasion of my privacy. By this time the strain was telling so much that I asked my GP to refer me back to the original psychiatrist. My GP tried but he refused to see me, instead arranging for me to see an alternative liaison psychiatrist in Bristol. I have continued to see this man since, initially largely as a result of the persuasion of my GP, and he has become a lifeline.

Eventually after six months the MPS gave the second assessor an ultimatum. Either come up with a report or her opinion would be discounted and I would see a new assessor. This finally provoked action and over a year from the initial referral I finally had sight of the two reports and the Health Screener's opinion.

The two reports were diametrically opposed, but even the second assessor was forced to admit that there was no evidence that I was a danger to patients. The Health Screener took the middle ground and suggested supervision, nominating the original referring psychiatrist. I refused, as after all he had refused to see me when I asked. So another individual was nominated and again I heard nothing. Eventually I phoned the nominated individual, catching him somewhat by surprise and he told me that he had told the GMC that he felt my case was too complicated and needed someone with a special interest. So again more waiting. Then finally a third nomination – a forensic psychiatrist. This just exemplified the feeling of being a criminal that the whole system engenders.

However, several years on we are contemplating the end of supervision after monthly sessions. My supervisor has moderated a meeting between myself and the original referring psychiatrist at which he apologised for the way in which he instituted the referral. I have ongoing contact with the liaison psychiatrist in Bristol and am in the initial stages of individual psychotherapy dealing with some of the traumatic issues of the past. I am working as a part-time GP and part-time academic and am undertaking a research degree. My mood has been reasonably stable on medication and I have had no extended periods of time off work. My friends and my GP have been a lifeline without which I would not have survived this far. Now, for the first time in years, I feel I am looking forward instead of back.

As to the GMC, initially I had nothing but anger for what transpired. Now when I get copies of the reports I still get angry, and sometimes I wonder about the future, about what future employers might think. It has certainly changed my career so far in that my training practice declined to have me as a partner when the senior partner (my trainer) retired, as I was then still in the midst of the initial process when the outcome was far from certain. However, I cannot honestly say that is something I regret . . . for now I have a balance, a life that suits me, and am even finally beginning to acknowledge that not all psychiatrists are evil. After all he only did what he thought was right and I'm not sure that I have the right to criticise that; the manner of it maybe (but for that he has apologised), but the actual act . . . for do we not all believe that the patient must come first? It's just that sometimes the doctor *is* the patient.

Chapter 9

Inside every doctor is a patient

Joanna Watson

During my psychiatric firms as a clinical student, I was appalled when I first heard doctors encouraging patients to like themselves. In Sunday school, I had learned that it was a Christian virtue to hate myself. I still practised this diligently. But the more I reflected on the psychiatric prescription, the more reasonable it seemed. I concluded that these crazy psychiatrists were right – 'love your neighbour as yourself' – and that there was something seriously wrong with my thinking, if not also with me.

My low self-esteem has an upside. The patient within me has always been willing to be open and honest about my difficulties and to seek local professional help. However, my not identifying with doctors who define themselves by their status has added to my isolation.

Given any kind of stress, I eat. My eating disorder began around O levels and developed insidiously. Whenever I felt bored, anxious or frustrated with revision, I would go to the kitchen for a slice of cake or cheese. By A levels, I was starting to respond to any uncomfortable emotion by eating. During my second year at Cambridge University, the year of the Cambridge rapist, I had my first binge: a large loaf of wholemeal bread wolfed down with margarine, marmalade and a pot of tea. My eating grew increasingly chaotic: the binges mushroomed: I became obese. I felt out of control, overwhelmed by unmanageable feelings – anger, sadness, fear, disgust, guilt, shame . . . I desperately wanted help but did not know where to turn. I thought that I was the only person in the world with this compulsion.

Compulsive overeating is still not formally recognised. Binge eating disorder had not yet been described. I gradually discovered that, among people with eating disorders, only thin and/or bulimic individuals were taken seriously. Consequently, I replaced simple bingeing with bingeing–starving; bingeing–purging; bingeing–dehydrating; and finally bingeing–vomiting (*Sublimia neovosa*, page 102). Over-concern about fat and, to a lesser extent, weight was a late entanglement, reinforced by treatment. Over 35 years, I have been many shapes and sizes (*In the moonlight*, page 101), once gaining 6½ stones in three months. At its nadir, life became one endless binge. I consumed up to my body weight of food each day and expelled what I could.

During my clinical training in London, I loved the contact with patients but dreaded the humiliating ward rounds and habitual exams. I felt overwhelmed by the amount that I needed to learn and inadequate for the task. During two periods of sick leave, first with anxiety and depression and later with glandular fever, two sets of contemporaries left me behind. The medical school was initially supportive, eager to dissuade me from giving up medicine. The subdean found me a tutor and lent me some sheet music of Saint-Saëns' *Le Cygne* 'to play until the sadness passes'.

As Cambridge finals approached, the support retreated during a series of attachments to peripheral hospitals. Every day for six months, I debated with myself whether I could face the pressurised revision, arbitrary assessment and uncertain outcome of taking finals. Paralysing panic alternated with my resolve to finish what I had begun. Doctors diagnosed my dizziness and abdominal discomfort as anxiety although these were not my usual symptoms. Stress did not explain an abnormal blood test result, eosinophilia. My conviction that we were missing something physical was dismissed as being 'just another neurosis'. Eventually, to my horror, I passed a segment of *Taenia saginata*. Purged of two metres of tapeworm, which I had probably acquired during my elective period in Kenya the previous year, I continued to stuff myself with food and facts. Weeks later, I qualified.

The Jungian psychotherapist whom I saw as a student would not take my bingeing seriously as a problem in itself but examined my past for causes. He belittled my memories of feeling suffocated. After manipulating my emotions over several years, he announced unexpectedly one session that this was our final meeting. Stunned, angry, impotent, I acquiesced.

Initiation as a house officer in the early 1980s meant a year of sleeplessness and powerlessness. During the first weekend of my surgical job, I worked continually from 07.00 on Friday taking routine bloods until the end of theatre at 22.00 on Monday: 87 hours without any sleep and only a half-hour lull on Sunday (*weekend on call*, page 97). The firm – consultant, registrar and house officer – failed to meet the General Medical Council requirement to provide full-time on-site registrar cover for pre-registration posts. The registrar spent half his time assisting the consultant at a private hospital, leaving me to make decisions beyond my professional competence. Despite pressure to collude, I raised my concerns with the consultant; the other consultants; the District Management Board; and finally with the General Medical Council. The job subsequently lost its recognition as a pre-registration post. That and helping several patients to give up smoking were the most useful things I did that year. For myself, I drew pictures of house officers committing suicide. I ticked off the last 140 days of my sentence on a chart. Then I gave up medicine.

I was uncertain what to do next. I had trained as a doctor to help people improve their health. I resolved not to return to medicine unless I found a job which threatened neither my health nor that of patients. Had flexible training been available for junior doctors, I would have explored general practice, neurology and cancer research. Although I had a longstanding interest in mental health, I recognised the dangers of training in psychiatry with unresolved problems of my own. In the following two and a half years, I faced the stigma and financial hardship of unemployment, with problems of structuring my time and finding a purpose for each day. I met contempt from former colleagues and friends for abandoning medicine.

During this period, I sought help for depression and bingeing. A weekly behaviour therapy group disregarded my eating habits. A compulsive overeating self-help group required excessive travelling. I then attended a community mental health centre five days a week for nine months. Most of the staff there were more familiar with the jargon than the principles of therapy. However, I learned what I could from Gestalt therapy, drama therapy, art therapy and other group work. To my face, the staff acknowledged my determination, positive contribution and willingness to take risks. Behind my back, they ridiculed me for using the word 'autonomy'. They ended all the groups with a fortnight's notice.

Later, I discovered community medicine, forerunner of public health medicine. I liked its broad perspective and holistic approach. I supported its emphasis on promoting health and preventing disease and disability. Being an independent voice for health resonated with my interest in neglected, unglamorous areas of need.

A consultant on an appointment committee recognised my abilities and potential despite my flawed *curriculum vitae*. She facilitated my introduction to community medicine by creating a special senior house officer post for me. Moving to be nearer my family, I then completed my postgraduate training in public health medicine, full-time and without any breaks, despite continuing health problems. Clinical psychology offered me too little, too infrequently, at a time when I was preoccupied with membership exams. Occasionally, I received Christian ministry and prayer, from sacraments to deliverance.

Throughout those years, I was an active member of a Christian group in my village sending food parcels to individuals in Romania. I 'adopted' a Romanian doctor and her family, offering what support I could; and visited the country twice during the most restrictive years of Ceauşescu's regime. After the revolution, the Romanian Ministry of Health invited me to work as a voluntary public health specialist at a centre for preventive medicine. Supported by selling my car, half-skeleton and other possessions and by charitable donations, I spent an intriguing two and a half years working in Romania.

I was 39 when I remembered my childhood sexual abuse. Remembering was both a shock and a relief. There is independent evidence corroborating some of my memories of abuse over 14 years by men and women. I suddenly understood why I had such low self-esteem and mistrust of my body. My memories of suffocating and my incapacitating fear of the Cambridge rapist made sense. But I needed some time out to recuperate.

The most consistent and constructive support that I have received since then has been from a psychiatrist specialising in eating disorders. He is sensible in both senses; and treats medically qualified patients as any others. He does not give up on patients, but now seems perplexed about how to help me disentangle myself from bulimia. The outpatient programme did not work for me. I then wanted to try inpatient treatment, although there was no specific programme for bulimia. In desperation, I had to emaciate myself; convince my psychiatrist that I wanted to get better, as I genuinely did; and wait for a bed on the anorexic unit.

I survived 15 weeks as a voluntary patient on an acute psychiatric ward in the mid-1990s (*Pyjama people*, page 98). The principles of the anorexic regime were asylum, uniformity and removing the burden of choice; there was no flexibility to meet bulimic or individual needs. Initially, I was confined to a single room and allowed two supervised baths a week. Being watched by a nurse while I bathed triggered memories of my abuse in bathrooms. Later, I had to share a dormitory with four anorexic patients and three televisions. My clothes were restricted to pyjamas. Therapy comprised one weekly session with my psychiatrist and another of art therapy. I spent my days observing, listening, reading and reflecting my experiences in poems, drawings, collages and needlepoint.

I enjoyed the food but found supervised meals with anorexic patients bizarre. There was an unspoken competition among them to be the last to finish eating within the time allowed. Instead of eye contact and conversation, local radio often accompanied the meals. For me, this irritating distraction was contrary to the principles for tackling overeating. We were weighed on Wednesdays and Sundays and expected to gain one kilogram a week. I gained ten kilograms in the first fortnight before the staff agreed to prescribe diuretics for my gross oedema.

I had no say in my treatment other than whether I stayed in hospital. My concerns about having a yeast infection or food intolerance were considered irrelevant and not worth investigating. Only my personal nurse appreciated the relevance of my requests for supervised eating in the canteen and body work therapy. With these needs unmet, I eventually discharged myself. Nine years on, I have still not been offered any cognitive behaviour therapy.

The most damaging incident that I experienced during therapy occurred at a rape and sexual abuse centre. Having formed a close therapeutic relationship with an experienced counsellor, I told the story of my abuse using words and artwork. Regression work triggered flashbacks, which the counsellor handled inappropriately. She later breached the professional code of ethics and practice by terminating my open-ended therapeutic contract without consulting me, informing me one evening by fax. She refused to return my personal writing and drawings, which we had agreed at the outset were my property. Shell-shocked but maintaining my dignity and integrity, I pursued a formal complaint until the financial and emotional costs became too great.

The counsellor had written that I needed a residential therapeutic community. My psychiatrist agreed with me that this would be detrimental to my recovery. I began to prepare to return to work.

Six years out of work with depression and fibromyalgia had set the odds against my returning to paid employment. I had lost skills, confidence and the habit of work. I wanted to work in academic public health. But I lacked the research experience that I needed to get a post to gain that experience. Being on the specialist register limited my options for retraining. However, a senior lecturer gave me a weekly session of unpaid therapeutic work. Supported by the occupational physician, the postgraduate dean later provided funding for my part-time retraining as a specialist registrar in public health. My determination, openness and a graduated programme of work helped me reintegrate into mainstream medicine.

My subsequent employment in a university department of epidemiology and public health has been precarious. Despite the need for more academic doctors, especially women, the Flexible Careers Scheme only covers clinical work. My career history and age make me an unlikely candidate for a research fellowship. Instead, I have worked as a part-time non-medical research associate on a series of short-term contracts (one to seven months). For 18 of the last 24 months, I have been retained on contracts for one hour of paid work a week while subsisting on income-based Jobseeker's Allowance and charitable gifts. Low self-esteem leaves me vulnerable to exploitation.

Unemployment does not provide the unlimited time that many overworked doctors imagine. Income subsides. Choice dwindles. Horizons shrink. Life becomes impoverished. Without opportunities to use my skills and creativity in meaningful ways, I become demotivated. The benefits system restricts the hours and type of voluntary work that one may do. Even minimal income from paid work may be financially disadvantageous if, for example, it makes one ineligible to receive free NHS prescriptions or full council tax benefit. Few professional bodies offer reduced subscriptions for doctors on benefits. This is the poverty trap within medicine.

Signing on can be a demeaning experience. Bureaucracy, depersonalisation and institutional suspicion pervade the Jobcentre Plus. Clients are potential abusers of the system. Staff are fallible processors of tedious paperwork. Cameras monitor both alike. The database of job vacancies is largely irrelevant for doctors. Few people outside medicine appreciate the nature and degree of specialisation within the profession. Given the shortage of doctors, an unemployed doctor raises awkward questions.

My professional and voluntary work over the past four years has included working with and for people with learning disabilities. I see this as my future vocation. My strengths and interests lie at the interface of academic and service work. I aim to use my skills in public health, epidemiology, research and writing to promote the health and quality of life of people with learning disabilities and their family carers. I plan to do a PhD on mental health problems in these groups. With the support of a local consultant in learning disability psychiatry, I have been accepted on the Flexible Careers Scheme for three years. I recently began work as a part-time associate specialist in learning disability psychiatry with a special interest in research. For the first time in my medical career, I feel valued both as a member of a supportive team and as a unique human being.

With a mustard grain of faith, I am becoming more than a survivor. Healing and forgiveness are processes. Autonomy, boundaries and control remain key themes for me. I am exploring new ways of dealing with here-and-now issues and developing a healthier lifestyle. My holistic approach to overcoming bulimia has uncovered intolerances to wheat and other foods, which probably arose from decades of overeating and previously impeded my recovery. During many locust-eaten years, I avoided music: it touches something too deep. Now, after a 23-year *tacet*, I am playing my oboe again, using it to express myself, meet people and discover life.

Chapter 10

Running on empty

Nikki Paiba

Doctors are in a high risk group for burn-out and major depression, but tend to think that it won't happen to them. However, many doctors do suffer with these sorts of debilitating illnesses. Unfortunately, I am one of them. The last few years of my life have been hell and I have been through an absolute nightmare.

I was a competent and respected junior doctor on a popular specialist registrar rotation. I had hoped that my working conditions would improve with time, but they didn't. I was still doing one in three rotas in an acute specialty where there was little time for much sleep. I felt awful but put it down to chronic sleep deprivation and stress. I was extremely unhappy and regularly drove to and from work in tears. I managed to cover up my unhappiness by smiling and pretending to be cheerful at work.

I felt overworked, undervalued and unappreciated. I spent all my time caring for others but no one cared for me. What other profession would allow some of its members to go without food or drink, two basic human necessities, on such a regular basis? I felt that I was being both physically and mentally tortured. I was existing just to go to work only to return home to work, because I had one last postgraduate exam to sit. I had sailed through previous exams, and was determined to push myself to keep going in order to achieve the final exam. I would then change my job in order to protect my sanity.

However, I began to feel more and more desperate. I started to have recurrent thoughts about wanting to go to sleep never to wake up again, and about cocktails of drugs and doses that I could use. I had no life. There was no point in being alive any longer.

Eventually, I couldn't hide the desperation any longer. I was found in a depressed state, by a colleague from a different specialty, who contacted the occupational health department. I found myself with an appointment with one of their doctors for the same day. I could no longer pretend or cover up my true feelings. I told him how desperate I was feeling. It was a relief that he seemed to understand, and a surprise that he was sympathetic too. However, I was shocked when he told me I was too depressed and too unwell to work. I felt guilty about not doing on-calls and letting my colleagues down, but he told me that he wouldn't allow me to return whilst I wasn't in a fit state to be at work.

Having been stopped from working, I collapsed into a heap and ground to a complete halt. I was absolutely burnt out. Frazzled with exhaustion, I wondered how my heart had the energy to pump blood around my body. I experienced marked biological symptoms of depression. For weeks I endured endless nights of insomnia. I was so tired but my distressed brain didn't know how to sleep anymore. Eventually I experienced auditory hallucinations. This frightened me so much that I agreed to try benzodiazepines, but doses escalated rapidly. With the help of a longer acting benzodiazepine, I eventually achieved some sleep, although it was dominated by numerous and very vivid nightmares during which I relived unpleasant parts of my past. I felt very nauseous and completely lost my appetite. I was amazed at how quickly two stones in weight just fell off me. This frightening process was eating me alive. I felt dazed and detached, and experienced intense feelings of depersonalisation. I felt so strange that my brain could have been made of porridge. I have felt incredibly sad and despondent, and I have cried inconsolably on occasions. Words cannot describe the despair and emotional torment.

In retrospect, I started to become progressively more depressed once I qualified and started working as a pre-registration house officer. I had struggled on for years thinking I was just tired, and had no idea that I was showing symptoms of depression which were becoming more severe with time. Although I am medically qualified, I did not realise I was becoming unwell, and I didn't appreciate how awful and frightening clinical depression could be, until I experienced it myself.

Unfortunately, many people, including some in the medical profession, still do not understand depression as an illness, and show prejudice and stigma towards those who suffer from it. The everyday use of the word 'depression' to mean 'feeling fed up' belittles clinical depression. It is a very real illness that is destructive, debilitating and frightening.

Over the last few years my life has completely fallen apart. I now have to pick up the pieces and rebuild my life. During the bad days, when I'm feeling particularly despondent, this seems like an impossible task. During the good days, I feel more positive and hope that I will manage to find a life that is worth living. The road to recovery is a long and stormy one, but I really want to get there.

Extracts of this article also appear in a personal view published in the *BMJ*: (2001) Why am I crying. *BMJ*. **323**: 1010.

Chapter 11

Since childhood

Petre Jones

I've wanted to be a doctor since childhood and now I work as a GP in East London, and am a GP Trainer and Course Organiser. Unfortunately, I have also had problems with depression since I was a child and now have a formal label of unipolar affective disorder.

My first episode of depression was at about age 8 or 9, but unsurprisingly it wasn't recognised at the time. Nor was it picked up at age 13 when I was getting intrusive suicidal thoughts. Every 2–4 years I've had an episode of major depression and managed to hide it very well, even from those most close to me. By the age of 35 I was still unlabelled, but with management responsibilities in chairing a large training practice, being a course organiser, chair of the GP co-op and various other projects and interests, I became depressed again. Rationalising away intrusive suicidal thoughts – honestly believing that everyone gets them, I started to self-medicate with antidepressants, which worked to begin with, until my supplies ran out. I felt better so didn't get any more, but dealing with paroxetine withdrawal effects was uncomfortable. Inevitably I became low again, and continued to work excessive hours with excessive responsibility to prop up my non-existent self-esteem.

Eventually, prompted by the prospect of an 'open and honest' practice away-day, my then practice manager took me to one side and asked me what was happening. I revealed a bit to her, but within a couple of days the flood gates opened and suicidal ideation was intense, as was de-realisation. I thought of using a pethidine injection overdose and raided the practice stock only to change my mind at the last minute and destroy the lot, except for one ampoule in case a patient needed it!

A couple of days later, between morning surgery and baby clinic, I rigged up a set-up to give myself an air embolism. My practice manager found me and the cat was out of the bag. There followed a whirlwind of BMJ counselling line, seeing my GP, seeing a psychiatrist, admission and more psychiatrists. I will never forget the fear on my wife's face as I was driven off to hospital.

Six months later, after two admissions (NHS funded to a private unit), loads of therapy, including 70 hours of CBT, and bucketloads of drugs (oh, and running a two-day residential course for my registrars!), I was ready to start part-time at work. The practice was really good at allowing me to gradually build up my workload, and I got back to full-time.

A little flexibility from my partners allowed me to keep going, having times of reduced workload when I had a wobble. I continued to see my psychiatrist, my CPN, my GP and took loads of medication.

The inevitable happened, however, three and a half years later when I had another major episode. This time I was self-harming, had paranoid thoughts about those around me and was very stiff and slow. I experienced de-realisation, hallucinations and would sit unmoving for hours. I was admitted again when I tried to stab myself with a scalpel and was scared my partners were coming to get me. I went to a local NHS unit and was put in a 'side room' that was little more than a cupboard with a bed, an ineffective light and a window made up of some glass, some scratched translucent plastic and hardboard. Not a perfect place to put anyone, let alone someone already deeply depressed.

A nightmare admission followed, with staff seemingly afraid to talk to me, let alone listen, and a psychiatrist who decided to label me as having a personality disorder, for no readily apparent reason. I discharged myself, and ended up being told to get treatment from another Trust, although the PCT haven't worked out yet if they can fund this. Writing a complaint letter ended with me only getting more damaged. I spent two peaceful weeks being watched and cared for by my parents. My CPN, the psychiatrist from my previous admission and my GP continued to see me and I slowly started to recover, and after a few months returned partially to work.

There is always a 'but' with this illness, and I found that my previous excessive workload and management role in the practice were no longer compatible with being healthy, and the practice was unable to be flexible enough to allow me to reduce it – I probably wouldn't have allowed myself to anyway, because of the impact on my self-esteem.

So I took the decision to leave and set up a smaller practice with a friend who was having childcare problems. It was either that or face a steady deterioration in health. I said to myself I could perhaps keep going for another two years. So, with encouragement from friends and professionals, I left the 'security' of a well established practice and plunged into the deep end to start a practice from scratch, with no patients. We did have a big grant from an urban regeneration corporation, and refurbished premises from the local housing association, but basically it was just the two of us.

Now, after an amazing year, we have a practice that works around close supportive teamwork. All the staff know my story and are happy to support me. My partner and I work so that I am flexible so she can work around childcare she is happy with, and she works around my mental health needs, offering support, some time off regularly, watching my workload and mental state, and not least building up a £20K contingency fund for when I'm next admitted, for locum costs etc. We are also a training practice, so registrars can see at first hand what we've done and why.

I live on with a severe mental health problem. I am now on lots of tablets, seeing CPN, psychiatrist and GP, and having psychotherapy at the Tavistock Clinic. But I also continue to be a full-time GP and educationalist. I have, for now, balanced my childhood dream with my childhood nightmare, and the key to this is flexibility in the workplace and having colleagues who are supportive and form a warm team, and professionals whom I respect and who respect me.

Chapter 12

Telling the story

Anon

I became depressed in the year 2000 as a result of life events. I was a second year psychiatry SHO at the time. I blamed how I felt on the effects of revising for part 1 exams but I continued to feel worse after passing part 1. It was not until my thoughts turned to suicide that I even realised that I was depressed. By then I was far from my normal active self and simply wanted to stay in bed on any pretext.

Having realised I was ill I started using self-help CBT techniques and sorted out the life problems that I believed caused my illness. I felt sure my low mood was reactive and with time and practical steps I would be fine.

Unfortunately, I just got worse and by Easter 2001 the suicidal planning was a frequent preoccupation. I realised I needed help, but how? I lived in the catchment area of my Trust and knew the juniors throughout the region from our Masters course. I was reluctant to see the GP as I was not over-impressed with them and I felt I had more than a primary care depression. I decided on the National Counselling Service for Sick Doctors. They were very helpful on the phone, giving me the numbers of two consultants just outside the region. Unfortunately, both consultants' secretaries said the psychiatrists were too busy for extra work. I rang the counselling service back and thay spoke with the secretaries and persuaded one of them to make me an appointment six weeks later. I was really disappointed, as taking into account the delay in benefit from antidepressants this meant it would be at least two months and probably nearer three before I felt any better. I reluctantly decided to go to my GP instead.

My GP gave me a brief consultation during which his only comment was 'fine, name your poison', so I chose an SSRI and he prescribed it and sent me on my way. By then I was desperate for some objective help as I just felt so awful and it was hard to maintain any perspective, but he left me feeling totally alone. The SSRI did not work so after three months it got changed to venlafaxine, with little effect.

Then in hot summer I started to have the feeling of knowing that I was not real and did not exist. I was becoming psychotic but it was actually a wonderful respite from the suicidal ideation. I had enough insight at that point to refer myself to a private consultant out of the area. It cost me a small fortune to see him weekly but he was very helpful. I continued working full-time with no on-call for about six weeks after that before I felt unable to continue and went off sick. My tutor was wonderful and arranged for me to be admitted to a small private unit out of the area.

Unfortunately, the care was atrocious and I got no better. I had a lot of doctor friends visit me and two who questioned my very bizarre management have received a lifetime ban from entering that clinic again. By Christmas concern about my deteriorating mental state and lack of coherent treatment was such that my tutor decided to forget confidentiality and arranged to admit me to our local private beds under the care of the senior consultant from where I worked.

By then I needed ECT but there were ongoing concerns about the resuscitation facilities in the local private hospital so they took me twice a week to the unit where I worked to administer ECT. I completed a course of 14 ECT in March 2002 and was restored to my old self, but with poor recollection of the previous year.

After remaining well at home for 10 weeks and having normal psychometric testing and occupational health clearance, I was allowed to return to work in the mornings. I had been off for nine months in total and was delighted to get back. Everyone was lovely and welcoming and supportive towards me. I called into the ECT suite to thank the team for taking care of me and they were very positive about me being back. I returned full-time after two months of mornings and then started on-call a month after that. Occupational health told the manager that I could not do whole weekends on call at my own request.

Since then I have become Section 12 approved and this spring I passed part 2. Not a bad achievement a year after a course of ECT!

I guess there are two key messages I have taken away. First, it is possible to get well and have a meaningful happy life, even after an impressive bout of mental illness. Not everyone becomes damaged. Sometimes we are made to feel that mentally ill doctors are damaged goods, or a time bomb to regard with caution, but this is neither helpful nor true.

Second, we need a pathway into high quality care. I wonder if I would have got so sick if I had been able to access proactive management as soon as I realised it was necessary. In my case special treatment had its special problems in a dodgy private clinic. For me it was worth sacrificing confidentiality and being treated as any other local patient but I have been extraordinarily lucky that the hospital staff have not made an issue of it. The balance of pros and cons in this respect may well be different for others.

Writing this story down has made me feel disappointed that at a time when energy and volition were in short supply I had to make such an effort to get the help I needed.

Chapter 13

The other side of the sheets: a special case?

Anon

Editor's Note: Unlike all the other stories in the book, this author tells of their experience in hospital with a 'physical' diagnosis. However, the emotions described are just the same for those with mental illness: the loss of dignity, the fear, the needing to help.

It is generally accepted that as a doctor if you are admitted to hospital you receive special attention – or is it?

I recount my experience, not going for sympathy, but to make the point that doctors are special patients.

I'll begin in the middle, since it wasn't until I was getting better that all this began to matter. In fact it was an idle comment from a visitor along the lines of 'I thought you'd be in a side room' that prompted me to examine my own distress.

Yes, I too thought I'd be in a side room. Almost immediately I chastised myself for the thought. What right had I to special treatment? I was no different from any other patient. But I was. This is not pride or snobbery, just fact. As a GP in the local area admitted to the local general hospital I was indeed different and no matter how hard I tried to behave like other patients I could not.

From the start I presented late with a list of differential diagnoses rather than symptoms. The potential treatment modified my symptoms. Fear of a laparotomy made the abdominal pain 'not too bad' or 'tolerable' rather than 'awful' or 'excruciating'. The nausea from metronidazole started as they wheeled the drip stand towards the bed.

Conscious of the overworked nurses, I ignored the fact that I'd had morphine, manoeuvred drip, no slippers, to find a toilet. Embarrassed and apologetic, I was found in a heap on the floor by the sink, pyjamas round my ankles. Despite running taps, I failed to perform and was scooped into a commode back to bed.

The night passed in morose tears and indescribably morbid fears. The morphine-induced dreams placed me in the mortuary watching my own post-mortem. Being awakened by a cardiac arrest in the next bay did nothing to reassure me.

If you ever catheterise someone, please take him or her to a side room. I lay like a pithed frog while two unidentified observers stood 'where they could see'. The curtains twitched as a head appeared, looking for sister. Then, and many times later, the only privacy I found was in closing my eyes.

But maybe once a doctor, always a doctor and I could not ignore my fellow patients. The lady in the corner had a subdural haemorrhage and I watched with alarm the automatic cuff record her increasing blood pressure. When the lady opposite vomited, I held her and gave her fresh tissues, to be told off for sitting on her bed by the nurse who eventually came. It was left to me to explain why this meant nil-by-mouth again. When the other two had their drains removed, my professional comments on the wounds were eagerly awaited.

Fear of meeting my own patients kept me prisoner in this six-bedded bay. Then MRSA threatened any early return to work. The drip tissued. It seemed everyone was too scared to re-site it. The delay meant that the next IV antibiotics and accompanying vomiting coincided with visitors. Whilst delighted that the passing of flatus was a step forward, I was mortified it should happen simultaneously with vomiting in front of all these people.

I cried, openly and copiously. I wanted to go home, to be alone. I needed to get away from work.

Sick doctors are special. Sick doctors in hospital need to be separated from other patients. This is not a 'perk' but a necessity for their recovery.

Chapter 14

Themes from the stories

Petre Jones

Having presented the personal stories it seems important to try to highlight some of the key issues that they raise. This is by its very nature a somewhat subjective process but I have tried to pick out issues that are common to several of the stories and then use quotes to try to illustrate, and give evidence for, what I mean.

The first thing to say is that we owe a lot to the generosity of the writers of these stories for publicly sharing intimate details of their lives in such an open way. Some have shared their secrets anonymously, for a variety of reasons, and we respect that, and some, myself included, are happy to be identified. One might wonder why anyone should choose to do this. One writer describes openness as the 'upside of low self-esteem' – if you value yourself very lowly your story itself has little value and is easy to give away. To balance this I hope all readers will feel compelled, as I am, to treat all these writings as precious and unique, just like the authors.

Another reason why people might be so open, and this is true for me, is that the illness and story itself have already been played out in the light of widespread knowledge. My diagnostic event occurred at work where I was an established GP and educationalist and within hours the practice were getting calls from all over the district asking about me. I had no real option of secrecy, and in fact I find openness and honesty about my background counters reticence in others and shame in me.

The main reason people have contributed, however, is that they believe in this book. They wish to generously share something of themselves with the readers in the hope that this will help to shed some light on what it is like for doctors who have mental illness, and perhaps help to break down stigma and promote treatment within the profession. Finally one might wonder if we are all narcissistic showmen and women drawing attention to our plight for psychological gain, and many of us with low self-esteem will already have asked ourselves this question. I will have to leave it to the readers to decide on this, but there are definitely easier ways to be self-promoting!

Theme 1: Mental illness need not be a bar to a medical career

A few years ago I was leading a residential course on our VTS and, as so often happens on these things, the subject of mentally ill doctors came up, and in particular whether they should have to leave GP partnerships. One of the newer

SHOs, who hadn't yet got to know me, felt that as mental illness affected the mind it must also affect the judgement and therefore anyone suffering such an illness could not function reliably as a doctor. He has now learned different things about mental health and has become a sensitive and sensible GP who can see beyond this simplistic 'all or nothing' approach. I would be happy for him to be my GP. However, as an SHO he was stating a view that seems to be quite widespread among doctors who haven't really thought about the issues yet. Put simply, this view states that a doctor who is mentally ill is either unfit for medicine or will sink into a sad decline of poor practice. On the day I was admitted for the first time to a psychiatric unit, I said to my GP that this would of course mean the end of my career. I didn't understand her disagreement; I had bought into the myth that mental illness stops you working as a doctor.

What can we learn from our stories? Clearly, some doctors continue to work and have 'successful' careers by conventional standards.

> I live on with a severe mental health problem. I am now on lots of tablets, seeing CPN, psychiatrist and GP, and having psychotherapy at the Tavistock Clinic. But I also continue to be a full-time GP and educationalist.

> I started believing in myself again and re-entered higher training, obtaining my CCST without difficulty and with excellent references. I even had time to do an MBA with the Open University – as well as having two children.

> I now hold the consultant post of my choice.

> I have now retrained as a GP and work part-time.

> Since then I have become Section 12 approved and this spring I passed part 2. Not a bad achievement a year after a course of ECT!

> I am working as a part-time GP and part-time academic and am undertaking a research degree.

Others have not been so fortunate.

> For 18 of the last 24 months, I have been retained on contracts for one hour of paid work a week. Without independent means, I subsist on income-based Jobseeker's Allowance and charitable gifts. Low self-esteem leaves me vulnerable to exploitation.

As one might expect, with a range of people and a range of conditions, there are a range of outcomes. The myth that you can't be a doctor if you are mentally ill is, however, shown to be false.

It is also clear from the stories that we are not just talking about mild illness, although in the Doctors' Support Network we have no sense of comparing 'severity' of illness. Burn-out and stress are important in medicine because of their frequency and the disability caused, but here we are talking about severe depression, near lethal suicide attempts and psychotic features. My own example of severe recurrent depression with suicide attempts and some psychotic features has not stopped me continuing my career as a GP partner and Lead Course Organiser.

Severe and enduring mental illness, especially the affective disorders and eating disorders, is not necessarily a bar to working in medicine. Those working in recruitment, retention, occupational health and GP partners should take note if we are to avoid wasting skilled people.

Theme 2: Shame and the myth of the invulnerable doctor

One of the strongest themes from the stories is that of shame. Several of the doctors describe hiding their illness from colleagues and even close family, sometimes for years.

> Doctors have a tremendous fear of mental health. There is the fear of peer criticism and the belief that doctors don't get ill.

> Every 2–4 years I've had an episode of major depression and managed to hide it very well, even from those most close to me. By the age of 35 I was still unlabelled.

> I managed to cover up my unhappiness by smiling and pretending to be cheerful at work.

> I realised I needed help, but how? I lived in the catchment area of my trust and knew the juniors throughout the region.

> I did not even have a GP at the time. I kept it a secret for a year, I felt so ashamed.

> I had got fairly good at hiding my deep despair and at the end of that year people knew I was struggling, but no one saw the suicide attempt coming.

The strong-looking, 'invulnerable' doctor may indeed be covering illness, and giving no real clues. The doctor next to you, or indeed you yourself, may be suffering, and yet offering up a façade of ordinariness and professionalism, and unless you ask, or are prepared to disclose, no one will ever find out. Perhaps our next theme casts some light on the causes of this.

Theme 3: Driven to work (too) hard

Anyone who has climbed the greasy pole to become a doctor is likely to be a hard-working, driven person. There is a strong theme in our stories about people being driven from within, and also being driven by the expectations of others.

> I had a strong perfectionist streak, found it impossible to say no to people, looked after everyone else and helped them with their problems and felt guilty if I did something purely for me.

> I felt there were huge expectations around my future career.

> Inevitably I became low again, and continued to work excessive hours with excessive responsibility to prop up my non-existent self-esteem.

> Many of the people I have worked with start off being supportive but when I needed time off the support often waned.

> At medical school you're pushed and pushed academically, but you don't mature emotionally.

> During my clinical training in London, I loved the patient contact but dreaded the humiliating ward rounds and habitual exams.

> I felt overworked, undervalued and unappreciated. I spent all my time caring for others but no one cared for me. What other profession would allow some of its members to go without food or drink, two basic human necessities, on such a regular basis? I felt that I was being both physically and mentally tortured.

> I felt guilty about not doing on-calls and letting my colleagues down.

> I met with contempt from former colleagues and friends for abandoning medicine.

None of this is really just about those of us with mental illness – these are issues prevalent throughout all branches of the profession – but it is easy to see how this can magnify the low self-esteem felt by those who are ill, or fear they may be, reinforcing that sense of shame and stigma.

Theme 4: Self-treatment and therapy

In a state of shame and fearing for one's health, some doctors self-medicate and try to do their own therapy. This clearly goes against GMS guidelines on self-treatment and, given the altered judgement of some of our ill doctors at the time of their illness, is clearly a bad idea.

> I started to self-medicate with antidepressants, which worked to begin with, until my supplies ran out after a few months.

> Having realised I was ill I started using self-help CBT techniques and sorted out the life problems that I believed caused my illness. I felt sure my low mood was reactive and with time and practical steps I would be fine.

Self-treatment presumably results from a combination of convenience, shame, and altered self-judgement and low self-esteem.

Theme 5: The health system causes problems because we are doctors

We know the rules of the health system, and the ways of working those rules to secure the best for our patients, but when it comes to us as patients it seems we face some unique problems because we are doctors. Issues about an under-resourced service that doesn't work for anyone are not really the same problem and I have not included them. In fact, our authors are remarkably forgiving about NHS resource limitations. This section is about the problems doctors face with the health system simply because we are doctors and so we don't quite fit as patients.

No GP

> I did not even have a GP at the time. I kept it a secret for a year, I felt so ashamed.

Doctors are notorious for not being registered with a GP, and this inevitably leads to loss of holistic care, the opportunity for the primary care team to deal with the doctor's health, and problems accessing secondary care in the conventional way. Continuity of care between episodes is also lost. It is easy to see why this should happen. After all, we can all treat minor and common illness and have easy access to drugs, but general practice offers us much more than this if we engage with it.

> Fortunately, I had a good GP who saw me regularly, until it became obvious I was having a major depressive episode.

We don't talk

> A nightmare admission followed, with staff seemingly afraid to talk to me, let alone listen.

> My GP gave me a brief consultation during which his only comment was 'fine, name your poison'.

It is hard for health professionals to deal with colleagues. It is embarrassing and breaches the usual rules of inter-colleague communication that protect our personal selves from our professional selves. So when I, as a GP course organiser, was being admitted by a locum SHO, I tried hard to give him the history he wanted, rather than honestly talk about what I felt was happening. This was a clear distortion. When on the ward the staff grade doctor asked me about lithium blood levels – where they had been done and when – but nothing on a more personal track. The GP in the second quote seems also to have been blocked from entering a more in-depth discussion. Friends and colleagues don't ask personal questions, but when the colleague is a patient, we must.

Odd care pathways

> I was found in a depressed state, by a colleague from a different specialty, who contacted the occupational health department. I found myself with an appointment with one of their doctors for the same day.

> Intervention by a work colleague meant I saw a consultant who visited me at home.

> I had enough insight at that point to refer myself to a private consultant out of the area.

> I wonder if I would have got so sick if I had been able to access proactive management as soon as I realised it was necessary.

> I was spared the weekly interrogation session (sorry, ward round) because of my status.

Entering the health system through unorthodox routes is bound to distort the delivery of care. Our health system is set up so that primary care is the first port of call, from which we can access secondary care, or the private health system. It is unusual for occupational health to be the first port of call, and this might have led to the protracted treatment phase for this doctor. Going straight to secondary and private care bypasses primary care in a way that can be unhelpful, especially for ongoing continuity. As the third quote suggests, proactive management at an early stage would be ideal and, at least in theory, primary care is the first port of call in this, except that the doctor who wrote that comment had a GP who didn't offer a helpful service! The final quote is interesting. The author sees this small dignity as positive, but one wonders about the impact on teamwork and the care plan.

It is not possible to say what real effects these unusual care pathways had. One could argue that patient-centred care for non-average patients will always lead to unusual solutions, but it may equally be true that if you bypass the usual care mechanisms you risk missing out such things as teamwork, communication and continuity.

Confidentiality

> Following the overdose I was admitted to the hospital I was working in. That was one of the all-time low points. The consultant I had worked for was covering that night, he came in and I remember him crying.

> So they took me twice a week to the unit where I worked to administer ECT.

> For me it was worth sacrificing confidentiality and being treated as any other local patient but I have been extraordinarily lucky that the hospital staff have not made an issue of it. The balance of pros and cons in this respect may well be different for others.

Reasonable confidentiality is a basic requirement of all civilised healthcare. How can the patient disclose personal stuff, behind the curtain of shame that shrouds mental illness, unless they can be assured that they can later return to their lives and put on again the layers of dignity that allow us to face the world and each other? You might think that this would be axiomatic for those looking after doctors, but, of course, as doctors we are part of the therapeutic community in which we work and can never get any sense of true confidentiality when being treated by doctors we know. Naturally, they will not discuss our details with others, but because the doctors, the OT, the nurses, the cleaners, are our colleagues and friends, the mere fact of them knowing about our illness and 'shame' means that we cannot ever return to the equal dignified working relationship there was before.

Being treated in our local hospitals is generally not appropriate. I was once sent a letter to come and do a section 3 assessment on a patient who was in the same hospital (different ward) that I was in at the time. Doctors should be offered treatment outside the area they work to maintain confidentiality and therefore emotional safety.

The GMC

> As to the GMC [Health screener procedures], initially I had nothing but anger for what transpired. Now when I get copies of the reports I still get angry.

> For do we not all believe that the patient must come first? It's just that sometimes the doctor *is* the patient.

The GMC, a unique part of the health set-up for doctors, is there to protect patients, and, in the case of sick doctors, to facilitate their access to treatment. Our one storyteller who had contact with them found it a prolonged and painful experience which seems neither to have protected patients nor to have helped the doctor. One cannot generalise from one person's experience, but it would be nice if the GMC could be seen as efficient and unbureaucratic in its dealing with ill doctors and remember that the doctor is the patient too in these cases. I am aware that the GMC is looking at the health system again and hope they can streamline the process. However, the idea of linking health issues with professional misconduct issues in one system seems to me to take us back to stigma and is unhelpful.

Theme 6: Glimpses of how the health service as a whole is adversely affecting all patients

Funding

> I discharged myself, and ended up being told to get treatment from another Trust, although the PCT haven't worked out yet if they can fund this.

> The funding for admission to the hospital where my psychiatrist worked had been taken away.

> Most mothers do not get admitted to a mother and baby unit.

The strange and sometimes seemingly arbitrary way in which decisions about service funding are made can disrupt care. For the first of these doctors there remains, after almost two years, some uncertainty as to which Trust would admit him if that were needed, and for the second, a change in funding arrangements meant not being able to maintain continuity of care. The shortage of mother and baby units, like adolescent units, is a national funding issue.

Poor standards of care

It is difficult in a resource-starved service to maintain proper clinical standards, so inevitably some care falls below what one would expect, but feedback to complain is not always easy. Our authors have been very gentle in their portrayal of poor standards of care, but we all know it happens in any large system.

> Clinical psychology offered me too little too infrequently.

> Regression work triggered flashbacks, which the counsellor handled inappropriately. She later breached the professional code of ethics and practice by terminating my open-ended therapeutic contract without consulting me, informing me one evening by fax.

> A nightmare admission followed, with staff seemingly afraid to talk to me, let alone listen, and a psychiatrist who decided to label me as having a personality disorder, for no readily apparent reason. I discharged myself, and ended up being told to get treatment from another Trust.

Damaging complaints procedures

> I pursued a formal complaint until the financial and emotional costs became too great.

> Writing a complaint letter ended with me only getting more damaged.

The complaints system is difficult to deal with even for well informed and articulate patients who work in the system; what must it be like for those less empowered than us?

Private care no guarantee of quality

> My tutor was wonderful and arranged for me to be admitted to a small private unit out of the area. Unfortunately, the care was atrocious.

> But there were ongoing concerns about the resuscitation facilities in the local private hospital.

These two comments are about the private sector, so presumably it is not all about resourcing.

Good care

> Four months in an NHS psychiatric unit got my medication the best it had been and the limited resources were stretched by committed staff to provide a reasonable service.

This comment about care being a function of the commitment of staff is really important. One wonders, though, how much more this unit would be able to provide if resources did not have to be stretched so far.

Theme 7: Flexible working

Now, after an amazing year, we have a practice that works around close supportive teamwork. All the staff know my story and are happy to support me. My partner and I work so that I am flexible so she can work around childcare she is happy with, and she works around my mental health needs, offering support, some time off regularly, watching my workload and mental state, and not least building up a £20K contingency fund for when I'm next admitted, for locum costs and hospital costs etc. We are also a training practice, so registrars can see at first hand what we've done and why.

The balance I have now seems to be working well, I work between two and a half and three and a half days per week as a long-term locum in a couple of local practices. I also do one clinic session in a cardiology clinic; this keeps up my interest in my favourite area of medicine.

I know many others in my position can not reorganise their lives in such a way that they continue to cope with stimulating yet stressful activities that are right for them while discarding the harmful stresses. Too many doctors find the system so inflexible that they have to leave medicine altogether. This is a sad loss for the individuals, the profession and society.

For now, I have a balance, a life that suits me.

Returned to work very gradually and was totally supervised as I did so.

Occupational health told the manager that I could not do whole weekends on call at my own request.

I was doing lab work. It meant I could organise my work around how I was feeling, doing repetitive lab work on days when I was having problems concentrating, and saving any reading for days when I had more energy.

I am now working as a part-time GP, which has made such a huge difference to the quality of my life that I can't begin to describe it.

Some of us have managed to find a balance between work and life within which we can function reasonably well. This has been achieved by accepting a degree of flexibility in the workplace to accommodate needs. It is heartening to see the level of flexibility that some of us have found possible, and of course one would like to see best practice rolled out across the country.

It took 15 months from discharge for me to pluck up the courage to work again – very limited as a returner to general practice.

For some of us that balance has not yet been achieved, either because of the disabling nature of the illness or because of the rigidity of institutional work patterns.

> As a flexible trainee in the hospital I have found you are treated as a
> second-class citizen. There is the attitude 'I wish I could have time off if
> I get stressed'. There is little appreciation that depression is not just
> feeling a little stressed.

> And I found that my previous excessive workload and management
> role in the practice were no longer compatible with being healthy, and
> the practice was unable to be flexible enough to allow me to reduce it –
> I probably wouldn't have allowed myself to anyway, because of the
> impact on my self-esteem.

> Despite trying very hard to renegotiate hours it seemed that the only
> solution was to resign and think again.

Negative attitudes to flexible working (back to the myth of the invulnerable
doctor) both from colleagues and from within ourselves (shame and the driven
doctor) sadly still exist. To be fair, for me the level of flexibility I needed, and in
the end achieved, were way beyond what you could expect a busy large practice
to easily deliver and so, although sad, my needing to find work elsewhere was
inevitable.

If flexibility is a way to retain skilled professionals, we really must look at ways
to encourage flexibility. The flexible training scheme run by the deaneries is now
well established, and the flexible career scheme, which allows GPs at least to work
a varying number of sessions per week as a salaried practitioner, is another
welcome move. This comes as new money from central government. However,
attitudes amongst Trusts and existing practitioners will need to change if we are
not to lose people with valuable skills from the workforce. It is no longer
acceptable to think of doctors who suffer mental illness as 'a financial liability'
or 'lazy' or 'inadequate'.

Theme 8: The need for support

It can come as no surprise that the need for human support is mentioned in our
stories, as John Donne wrote: 'No man is an island, entire of itself'. We all need
the support and encouragement of others and it comes as no surprise either that
when this is lacking, our writers, already vulnerable, found difficulties.

> Mental illness was always a taboo subject in my family.

> I had lost touch with many friends.

> Many of the people I have worked with start off being supportive but
> when I needed time off the support often waned.

On the other hand when human support was present it was found to be
encouraging and empowering.

> I have also discovered the importance of a social support network, and
> of having at least one good friend who will give hugs with no questions
> asked.

I am very lucky that my husband, GP and work colleagues have been so supportive, insightful and understanding.

I have had a lot of support from my husband, flat-mates and certain friends, without which I would have committed suicide.

So, with encouragement from friends and professionals I left the 'security' of a well established practice.

It is appropriate to end this chapter on the theme that positive human interaction can help to restore our humanity. This is not just about mental illness, but about all of us as people. Building friendships, listening to each other and offering a shoulder to cry on is something we can all do, and can transcend the constrictions of our usual rules of interacting, for the good of all.

Summary

- Mental illness need not be a bar to working as a doctor.
- The invulnerable doctor is a myth that leads to shame and denial of problems.
- We drive ourselves to work (too) hard.
- Self-diagnosis and self-treatment is a bad idea.
- The health system causes doctor patients special problems.
- Problems within the health service cause different problems to all patients.
- Flexible working is helpful for sick doctors.
- Everyone needs human contact and support, especially when ill.

Chapter 15

Issues in treatment

Petre Jones

We have looked at many stories of doctors with mental illness and drawn out the common themes that arise. In this chapter we will look at specific treatment issues that arise.

None of our group feel that doctors should be treated differently just because they are doctors and therefore have some 'right to better treatment because of status'. Many of our group have low self-esteem, so according ourselves any status at all feels uncomfortable. However, all doctors know, or should know, that patients need to be treated according to their particular needs. So a hand surgeon will treat an injury in a violinist differently from one in a psychiatrist, and the treatment for a cataract becomes suddenly different when the other eye is glass.

The thoughts on treatment in this chapter are based on the obvious fact that doctor patients have unique needs which must be considered in making plans. Each of us will have different needs, but in this chapter we will look at the shared needs that all doctors as patients bring.

Stigma and confidentiality

> 1   It should be routine that doctors needing admission should be offered *admission to a hospital they do not work in* or, for GPs, refer to.

Although the professions looking after the sick doctor may keep strictly to the rules of confidentiality, the mere fact that a group of local colleagues is discovering intimate details about the sick doctor puts the doctor in a vulnerable position which will then compromise his future working relationships. Realising this, the sick doctor may either become more acutely aware of their vulnerability and feel humiliated, or may refrain from disclosing details to the healthcare team. Neither is in anyone's interest. Admissions to other units may be fairly easy in urban areas but even in remote areas of Scotland, say, admission away from home is possible. Of course, the downside of remote admission of course is that family and friends may find visiting difficult and this will impact on support networks after discharge. My experience of being 'admitted' 60 miles from home was that people were still keen to visit. One friend travelled one evening on public transport only knowing the name of the town she was heading for, with no idea of address or location. She got there in the end.

What of the idea of the special unit for health professionals that was piloted in the early 1990 by Dr Connolly at the Maudsley Hospital in London? They found that the range of illness was the same as in the general mentally ill population and funding for it was stopped. However, it did provide a unit where health professionals could go and not fear loss of confidentiality, it being an 'out of area team', and where staff would not be disempowered by caring for a doctor. On the downside such units were never likely to receive sufficient mainstream funding given the huge scale of the problem, and geographical distance to get to a unit would also be a significant issue for many.

This has left us with the traditional care pattern of commissioners of care, usually PCTs, making choices about places of admission on an ad hoc basis, but preferably not to Trusts where the doctor works. Currently this system doesn't work well. Some doctors have still been admitted to their own Trust, and others have subjected their GP or psychiatrist to long series of phone calls to negotiate a more appropriate place of admission in the midst of an emergency. Whatever the intentions of senior commissioners and Trust officers, the final decision on the day may rest with a member of staff who does not fully appreciate the particular needs of doctors as users of mental health services. All PCTs will face the problem of a health professional needing mental healthcare as an outpatient and, more importantly from our stories, for emergency admission.

> 2 All PCT commissioners need, as a matter of urgency, to put in place standing contingency orders in advance, so that any doctor needing admission can have access to a Trust outside their area, automatically.

This would not be a difficult thing to put in place, and the cost implications would not be great given that the need for admission had already been decided upon. This is an urgent need for action by all PCTs.

Stigma and access

This is about how the stigma of mental illness leads us to access care in unhelpful ways.

Self-prescribing is not a good idea. No one would argue with this. I self-prescribed paroxetine for three months without anyone knowing (I used tablets patients had returned) and it made my problems worse by masking them enough for me to get significantly sicker before I was properly treated. However, where does the boundary of appropriateness lie? Few would have a problem with prescribing an asthma inhaler to your child if you are away on holiday, for example, and what then is the difference between doing this for your child and doing it for yourself? Certainly if this became anything like routine you would lose continuity of care (unless perhaps you obsessively inform your GP of each and every such event), but you will gain a lot in terms of convenience. So what is different about drugs with a CNS action? The answer is simply insight. With a physical illness in your child you have a good idea what you can and can't do, and when judgement is being clouded by a parental relationship one can usually tell.

When my son, then aged 12 months, had his first anaphylaxis episode in the back of the car, I was able to give him adrenalin and chlorpheniramine from my on-call drugs box. I knew I was somewhat clouded (terrified!) at this point and went to A&E where one of my GP SHO's took over his care, and I became the worried parent. That was clear-cut, he was treated properly, and I behaved as a parent. Similar role changes are usually easy with one's own physical health. However, with mental illness things are very different. We lose insight – not always, of course, but sometimes – and the trouble is that if your insight is clouded you will not realise it because you have clouded insight! You cannot judge the severity of your own depression. When I self-medicated I judged my depression as mild to moderate, partly because if it had been severe I would have seen myself as worthless and unloveable. The action of grading my depression came up against my own cognitive distortions and defences which were caused by, or the cause of, the depression. My judgement was wrong. And if you won't know those occasional times when you have clouded insight you can never trust those times when you think your insight is fine.

> 3   Self-medication is a bad move on most occasions but must never happen at all, ever, for anything to do with your stress levels, mind, sleep or anything else CNS.

Another good reason to avoid self-treatment is that, as we have seen, human support is an important part of treatment, and self-medicating reinforces the withdrawal from others that is so common in mental illness.

Getting into the system

So, if we are not trying to treat ourselves, how do we best get appropriate treatment? The first part of this is having people around who will help us. Someone needs to be able to ask the hard questions. Too often someone in a team is seen to be struggling but no one picks it up, or enquires about it. We generally lack a culture of teamwork and mutual responsibility across the profession, and this may lead to a situation akin to Michael Balint's collusion or anonymity, where the person in the middle clearly has a problem, but it's a bit of a hot potato. As a result those professionals who could at least start to address the problem instead decline to take any responsibility, in the hope that someone else will deal with it.

> 4   What is needed is for all of us to be prepared to ask colleagues who seem to be struggling what is happening for them, and be prepared to listen to the answers.

Of course, when all else fails it must fall to the senior doctor in the team, consultant or managing partner to take the lead on this. For me, it was a skilled practice manager who first took the risk, sat me down with a drink and a sandwich and simply asked me what was going on inside me, and the hiding stopped and the possibility of help began. If in medicine there were a culture of true teamwork rather than the all too common rivalries and overtired, over-stressed people with barely enough emotional reserve to keep themselves going, let alone consider other people, it would be easier to stop those who were getting into real trouble.

Having been identified, general practice is usually the first point of access to the healthcare system. This does depend on us all being registered with a GP, of course. Many of us don't, it seems. It's embarrassing to go to a GP and be vulnerable, and we may well feel we know more about our health issues than the GP anyway. That is not the point. The GP is a point of access to objective healthcare, and provides a space to deal exclusively with your health issues.

> 5   Practices, training schemes and rotations and occupational health departments all have opportunities to remind doctors of the need to register with GPs. We should take these opportunities.

Occupational health in our writers seems to come off reasonably well. Confusion about what is disclosed to whom is an issue, but it seems that information is generally dealt with appropriately. However, in the context of this chapter one must remember that occupational health is not a treatment service, nor is it generally a point of access to secondary care.

> 6   On the other hand, occupational health is an important point at which the initial questions and identification of doctors in trouble can take place. This does require everyone to take the health screening process seriously.

Hopefully, stories of large numbers of doctors lining up to be screened by someone sitting at an open desk, in easy earshot of the next one in the queue, can be a thing of the past.

> 7   It is indefensible that for doctors in general practice there is still no effective occupational health service.

Counselling lines run by local organisations, BMA and DSN do exist, of course, but these generally provide a service to those who are identified or can identify themselves, which is not the same role.

Deanery recruitment

Deaneries often come across doctors experiencing troubles. In the complex transitions of the training process, and in the stress of the recruitment merry-go-round, issues regularly come to the fore. In my role in recruitment I have more than once come across colleagues I have been concerned for.

> 8   In all the machinery of recruitment there should be a process whereby these people are identified and followed up by a senior member of the deanery.

Equally, in the all too common scenario of a training grade doctor getting into trouble, we need to ensure that either a robust mentoring process is in place or that clinical tutors and their college tutors, and course organisers, feel it is their job to take a lead in supporting and guiding them. Of course, trainees may be wary of disclosing stuff to senior colleagues who may have a hand in their future career prospects.

Services such as the MedNet service in London Deanery are to be encouraged. MedNet is a very confidential assessment process run by The Portman Clinic and funded by the London Deanery. It provides for doctors to have a six-session psychoanalytical assessment undertaken by a consultant psychoanalyst. Only the analyst and his administrative assistant will know the name of the doctor, who is identified by number. I have been through this process and can strongly recommend it. Other deaneries should consider similar local solutions.

Treating doctor patients

It seems that many of us still seek help through the quick consultation in the corridor, either from GPs or secondary care colleagues. Perhaps this is less embarrassing – you're less likely to be examined! – or perhaps we want to retain some control. However, as I tell my 'extra' patients who want to talk about three long-term problems at once, off-the-cuff medicine does not work.

> 9   Make a proper appointment, with enough time, in the correct setting. Corridor consulting can lead to missed diagnoses, over-investigation, under-investigation etc. Don't do it.

> 10   From the GP point of view there is a need to understand something of the difficulty that colleagues have in consulting us, and treat each such episode as a potentially high risk consultation and look beyond the obvious to the deeper agendas, perhaps in a similar way to the way one might particularly look out for emotional issues in a postnatal examination.

These are the basic skills of general practice consulting and we need to be better at it. These are skills that can be learned and improved on. They are taught on all VTS courses but should be built in throughout one's career.

GPs also need to be aware of the mental health problems that are common in doctors, and this, of course, is one of the purposes of this book.

Once identified it is fair to say that any doctor with possible mental health problems is likely to present a complex set of problems. Because of this it is unreasonable on both doctor and patient to ask someone with limited experience to do the assessment.

> 11   Doctor patients are difficult and should be assessed by a senior clinician as soon as possible.

On one admission to hospital I was seen initially by a locum SHO, which was fine for the routine late-night question asking, but then not seen by anyone else until the consultant saw me two days later. This is not appropriate care. On other admissions I have been seen initially by the junior on call but by an experienced consultant within 24 hours.

Most doctors with mental illness do seem to get back to some sort of work, although often not medical work. Barriers to returning to work are often the prejudicial practices endemic in medicine and a lack of flexible working.

> 12   The Department of Health document *Mental Health and Employment in the NHS* contains many recommendations to make it easier for people with mental illness to be rehabilitated back into work. One wonders how long it will be before good intentions become common reality.

These 12 recommendations arise directly out of the experiences of our writers. They do not pretend to be the universal answer to all the issues of mentally ill doctors but anyone attempting to deal with the issues would do well to consider these seriously, as they arise from the real life expertise of those with first-hand knowledge.

Summary

- Doctors should not be admitted to the hospital they work in or, for GPs, refer to.
- PCTs should have emergency plans in place for doctors to be admitted to a suitable hospital when needed.
- Self-management should not happen.
- We must all be prepared to ask colleagues how they are, and be prepared to listen to the answer.
- We should take every opportunity to remind colleagues to register with an independent GP.
- Occupational health screening should be taken seriously.
- General practice needs a full occupational health service.

- The recruitment processes should include a mechanism for candidates identified as struggling to be referred to a senior member of the deanery.
- All consultations with doctors should be seen as potentially high risk and complex.
- Doctor patients should be seen quickly and assessed by senior colleagues.
- DoH recommendations in *Mental Health and Employment* should be implemented as soon as possible.

Part Two

What's It Like?

Chapter 16

Stigma and discrimination

Lizzie Miller and Petre Jones

Some examples of prejudice from within the profession

As an established GP I am less professionally vulnerable to prejudiced attitudes than some of my ill colleagues, and it is therefore possible for me to speak up about specific situations.

Why should I wish to write about episodes of prejudice? Doctors are after all human, and not perfect, so why focus on the failings of some of us? We talk a lot about the stigma of mental illness and the prejudice this fuels, but unless we can demonstrate real life examples, it will remain as an abstract evil and therefore can easily be ignored. So, here are three examples from the last couple of years which, although they didn't adversely affect my career, were very difficult to deal with.

First, take the example of doctor A, a senior local GP. She is respected for her high level of clinical care and the work she does as a member of the PCT Executive Committee. I have known her for many years as an energetic and effective doctor, the sort that I might have once hoped to be. She is the managing partner of a large practice which at the time was looking for a salaried GP. I was trying to set up a new small practice to make it easier to deal with my health problems.

During a conversation with a colleague, Dr A commented: 'I wouldn't touch a partnership with Petre with a barge pole . . . [because of his illness] . . . he's a total financial liability'.

In fact in my previous practice I had taken the lead on financial negotiations that had effectively increased partners' profits by 60% in one year, the locum costs of my past work absences had been covered by insurance and PCT reimbursement, and in our new practice we earn as much as at the old practice on a smaller workload. No practice I've ever been at has suffered financially, or in service development terms, because of my illness, and because of my tendency to overwork to boost low self-esteem, they have all done quite well.

So Dr A's comment was factually wrong, but of course is based on the premise that sick, particularly mentally sick, doctors are bad news. They leave you to do the work and cost you money. We are all sick from time to time and the future for us all remains unknown, so if Dr A sticks to her preconceived ideas it may take her a long time to recruit a doctor who is never ill and will only ever bring good things to the practice. Her prejudice is doing her no favours.

My respect for Dr A dropped a bit, although she remains an energetic and effective GP.

The second example concerns Dr B. He was a GP registrar living outside London who was thinking ahead to get a salaried job at the end of his training. We had a PMS growth-funded job available and Dr B seemed to fit the job well. In particular the job included some educational input to help the doctor gain MRCGP, which Dr B wanted to do. It all seemed to fit and Dr B accepted the offer after a suitable application process.

However, as the job got nearer he began to get cold feet. The smokescreen reasons were that the money wasn't quite enough and London is a horrible place. Both may be true but they weren't any better when he accepted the post.

The real reasons were eventually revealed. First, because of my illness, he felt that any tutorial or supervision sessions I undertook with him would turn into difficult sessions of me talking about and gaining support with my illness. Presumably the idea behind this is that mentally ill doctors spend all their time talking about their illness and can't do anything else. As an educationalist I find it quite insulting to suggest that I don't know the difference between a tutorial and a counselling session. Illness is a part of who I am, but, like any human being, I can never be defined by just one characteristic. I am also a trainer, a husband, a father, a driver, a runner etc.

The second reason was more upsetting. He had decided that I had a personality disorder (subtype not specified) and therefore would create problems for anyone around me. ICD-10 and DSMIV do define personality disorder, in quite careful terms, but we all know that PD is often used as medical shorthand for 'I don't like this person'. The underlying prejudice here is to do with finding mental illness threatening or difficult, creating a feeling of irrational personal challenge. Dr B's comments are revealed as baseless because I don't have what could be called a disordered personality, meeting none of the ICD-10 or DSMIV diagnostic criteria.

We told Dr B that we would not appoint him.

The third example is very GP-specific. Partnership deeds are the legal documents that partners draw up to govern the relationship between them. They are a bit like contracts but vary a lot between partnerships in the clauses they contain. In my last practice, 13 years ago, I signed such a deed which included a clause which said that in the event of a partner being detained under a section of the Mental Health Act 1983, the other partners could expel him from the partnership, and effectively sack them. I took no notice of the clause at the time. I still thought of myself as mentally well, and the deed was drawn up by competent medical solicitors. Other members of the group tell me that their deeds include such a clause, and it seems it was a common part of many older deeds. It was put in alongside the usual provisions for sickness absence and retirement from the practice on the grounds of ill health and absence from work for prolonged periods. The Mental Health Act clause was specific to mental illness. I am not aware of any deeds that included clauses to say that if a partner was admitted to intensive care or coronary care they would be expelled from the partnership.

So why the focus on mental health? The underlying prejudice seems to be the belief that doctors who suffer from a severe mental illness, as opposed to a 'physical' illness, will not get better, are going to damage the practice, need to be got rid of, and that this is a legitimate and reasonable thing to do. One need only look at the section of personal stories to see that this is not true, and certainly not fair.

It is unlikely that these discriminatory clauses could ever now be enforced given the Disability Discrimination Act, but the fact that they remain in deeds is unsettling, and can put undue pressure on ill GP partners.

To their credit, when I pointed out the clause in our deeds to my then partners they all agreed that it should be struck out of our deed immediately.

Prejudice is evil, because it takes preconceived negative ideas that have no basis in fact and applies them in a blanket way to people who just happen to have a particular characteristic, regardless of their circumstances or strengths. In that sense it is fundamentally dehumanising to us all, making both perpetrator and victim answerable to a meaningless myth. We must strive to stamp out all prejudice in medicine, and in this context, prejudice about mental illness in professionals. As mentioned above, it has already been a significant cause of one colleague's death.

Evidence for stigma

Doctors are rarely known for their radical views, so when we learn that 30% of the population believe mental health patients are dangerous and should pull themselves together[1] it is likely that a fair number of doctors share those opinions. There is very little research into doctors' beliefs and attitudes, even though 40% of mental health patients believe themselves to be discriminated against on account of their illness. What there is suggests that doctors, like the public, tend to blame their patients for their condition. It is important that we know what attitudes we are propagating, thus appropriate further research is important.

Anecdotal experience provides limited if sometimes worrying evidence. After my first episode of illness, my reference said (unbeknownst to be me), 'This doctor should never practise medicine again'. Admittedly that was almost 20 years ago. Comments such as 'I hope you are now over the problems you had when you worked with us previously' can easily be taken the wrong way. It does not help to be viewed as delicate or fragile, whereas being treated as normal does.

Experience in the Doctors' Support Network (DSN) shows that discrimination frequently involves other people deciding what you are capable of and what you are not. For example, regardless of their specialty, many doctors have been told that they should consider a less stressful specialty than the one they are currently training in. Doing interesting enjoyable work is not stressful. Retraining in another specialty is stressful and losing the opportunity to use specialised clinical skills is demoralising. It may be necessary to reduce working hours and adopt a more flexible approach to training. Nonetheless, illness in itself is not necessarily a reason to change career paths.

Blurred boundaries

Discrimination also stems from the tendency of doctors to blur the boundaries between health and capability. As doctors we use our medical knowledge and judgement to make decisions for patients. It requires a deliberate effort on the part of the doctor to avoid using the medical method to assess our judging colleagues, peers and juniors.

Members of the DSN have frequently experienced the results of this blurring of boundaries. At worst, consultants have taken junior doctors' medical notes to consultants' meetings to discuss a doctor's future clinical career. Such occurrences are hopefully increasingly rare. In other cases clinical supervisors proffer a combination of clinical, career and medical advice. Application forms often request personal medical details and revalidation includes a health question. These medical details are relevant to work only through the filter of occupational health. Clinical confidentiality applies to doctor patients as much as any other patient.

The GMC is perhaps the worst offender. The GMC uses similar procedures to assess health, conduct and performance.[2] This resembles the Civil Aviation Authority taking upon itself to decide whether a pilot was physically fit to fly a plane. Health is a matter between patients and their doctor, not for tribunals to decide. Occupational health physicians are trained to determine whether an individual is fit to do the job they are employed to do.

Thus a combination of unhelpful attitudes and failure to separate an individual's health from their working capability leads to discrimination against colleagues with mental health problems.

Possibly one third of doctors with mental health problems do not return to work after their illness and a further third work at below their capacity. Lack of support is frequently cited, and it is difficult to get back to work once the GMC are involved (source: survey membership of DSN – unpublished).

On a scientific level, negative attitudes to mental health have at least two significant effects. Many students start their medical careers with the intention of becoming psychiatrists. There is some evidence that the attitudes they are exposed to in medical school and on the wards lead to them changing their minds. It is also likely that negative attitudes tarnish research into mental health. It is safer to keep patients at a distance, pursuing a drug-based 'medical' approach instead of developing a challenging social psychological model of mental health and illness.

Tackling stigma and discrimination

Attitudes change through education and experience. Journals can be encouraged to carry articles about mental health, particularly those written by people with direct experience of mental illness. The Royal College of Psychiatrists Changing Minds[3] campaign has done a massive amount to alert society and the medical profession to the extent and effects of the stigma of discrimination around mental health. The government, Department of Health, GMC and BMA need to make an equal commitment. As influential members of society, we, as doctors, have a duty to clean up our own act at the same time as we expect society to become less prejudiced towards our patients.

We need to create firm boundaries between an individual's health and their ability to do a job. This includes removing questions about health from application forms and from the revalidation process. A strong occupational health service will serve to identify, support and rehabilitate the sick doctor. This approach will encourage doctors to seek help where necessary, instead of feeling forced to hide their illness for fear of losing their job or being referred to the GMC. This can be supported by other measures including looking at the special requirements of doctors as patients, the need for out-of-area referrals, rehabilitation schemes and flexibility in the workplace.

The legal framework to reduce discrimination exists. The Disability Discrimination Act protects individuals from discrimination on the grounds of mental or physical disability. It obliges the employer to make appropriate modifications to a job so that a disabled person can compete on equal terms with an able bodied employee. This can include altering or reducing a doctor's hours where such commitments might damage a doctor's mental health. The GMC states that the attributes of the independent practitioner include the maintenance of attitudes and conduct appropriate to a high level of professional practice. This includes a duty of self-awareness and insight into his or her own attitudes and temperament.

However, in isolation neither the law nor regulation can remove stigma from within a culture. This requires personal and organisational commitment. Language is important. Medical culture may allow us to describe people on antidepressants as wimps, but apply that comment to someone of a specific religion or race and it is easy to see how inappropriate it is. Doctors with mental health problems already feel deeply ashamed of their condition and to blame for their illness. Medical culture must stop reinforcing such self-destructive beliefs.

Support structures can help put stigmatising attitudes into context. The Doctors' Support Line (0870 765 0001) and Doctors' Support Network reassure doctors with mental health problems that they are not alone, and that there is a light at the end of the tunnel. Mental illness does not respect social class or specialty. It has a high casualty rate. If large numbers of doctors are not to be lost from the profession, if we do not learn to be kinder to ourselves and each other, there will be a bleak future for those who remain.

Finally, those of us who have been through the mill can help by presenting our condition in a positive light. Most people rely on stereotypes, which can be changed when challenged. Doctors learn their attitudes to mental health from those around them. If you can reject the prejudices and stigma within yourself and put your condition forward as part of the rich tapestry of human experience, it may be possible to engender compassion as well as curiosity in those who lead less troubled lives.

References

1 Crisp AH, Gelder MG, Rix S, Meltzer HI and Rowlands OJ (2000) Stigmatisation of people with mental illnesses. *British Journal of Psychiatry*. **177**: 4–7.

2   Brewer B (2003) GMC health procedures. *BMJ*. **326**: S106.
3   Royal College of Psychiatrists (2001) *Mental Illness: stigmatization and discrimination within the medical profession.* Council Report CR91.

Summary

- Stigma and discrimination against mental illness is endemic and common in the medical profession, from the GMC downwards.
- The legal framework exists to combat discrimination.
- Prejudice is common.
- Ill doctors tend to hide problems because of shame and stigma, which reinforces prejudice.
- Entrenched attitudes within the profession need to change.

Chapter 17

Easily misunderstood experiences

Petre Jones and Fiona Donnolly

As doctors who have experienced mental illness, we have been through episodes that are strange and perhaps hard to understand. We have found that some of the signs and symptoms of mental illness can be misinterpreted, and so we offer these examples and what they felt like from the inside in order to try to make the experiences more understandable. Perhaps this will give a little more insight into the troubled brain and what it is like to be inside one.

Disconnecting with the outer and inner worlds

Symptoms relating to internal and external disconnectedness are common. I have divided this section into symptom groups that reflect the differing degrees of disconnectedness experienced.

Psychodynamic disconnections

Like all of us, people with mental illness are prey to all the common psychological defences and cognitive distortions – the mind plays tricks. Just because we are ill does not mean our minds can't screw us up further too. Denial is perfectly normal and common, but when one of our group was in denial about having a chemical hepatitis, despite ample physical evidence, it became for a while impossible for her carers to treat her. Equally I have had the experience of, quite unintentionally, behaving selfishly towards a close friend, only finally noticing it long after her subtle cues had passed me by and she was literally shouting it out aloud at me. I was absorbed in difficult stuff at the time and completely blanked out her messages, because of course it was too painful for me to hear that I had hurt a friend.

Cognitive distortions are a bit more subtle but just as normal and just as difficult to deal with. When I was first admitted to hospital with depression, in the middle of the night, I remember seeing the large heavy lock on the front door to the hospital. This triggered for me an automatic thought about not ever being able to get out, and triggered a high degree of anxiety and distress. Of course I knew that people with depression were not locked up for ever anymore, but my mind, triggered by the sight of the lock, disconnected from the evidence and my own internal reality and freewheeled into an anxiety-fuelled catastrophisation (making things far worse in my mind than they were in reality). A similar reaction whilst being interviewed by a consultant psychiatrist led to a bizarre and erroneous label of personality disorder! Other cognitive distortions, like fortune telling and personalisation, are common enough in 'normal' people, but are more common in mental illness. They are normal ways for our minds to disconnect with objective reality, and make mental illness worse if you happen to be suffering from it at the time. There is no time in this book to go into detail about these psychological reactions and disconnections, but suffice to say they happen in spades in the mentally ill. They are a cause of a lot of distress, and may complicate diagnosis. They can however be challenged using cognitive behaviour therapy, skills present even in people with psychotic illness.

De-realisation

A commonly described symptom, especially in those suffering from depression, although also described in those suffering form a primary eating disorder. The feeling is one of being distanced from or separate from the world, so that people use terms such as 'being in a goldfish bowl', or 'feeling there is an invisible barrier between me and the world'. One person even describes meeting a friend and feeling they were 'peering in' to talk to them. This is usually not too distressing, but is very odd and can contribute to withdrawal, and the desire to simply curl up and hide. However, for some the experience is very distressing and can lead to self-harming simply to cause and experience pain to remind oneself that things are still real.

Bizarre stuff with some insight

Sometimes mental illness leads to us having bizarre thoughts and experiences that don't have any basis in reality and yet, strangely, at some level, we retain an ability at least in part to comprehend that these experiences are not real. For example, I once was sitting in a consulting room surrounded by the mass of computer equipment that is now indispensable to general practice. I was ill at the time and had a short-lived experience in which I knew that the computer wires were a threat to my safety as they would wrap themselves around my neck and strangle me. This was a frightening perception that fortunately only lasted a few minutes, and the wires reverted to normal innocent computer wires. However, with a little medical knowledge, although this had never happened to me before, I realised that this was some sort of psychotic-type experience and my irrational fear of wires was quickly replaced by a very rational fear that I was rather more ill than I thought. Realising that you are significantly mentally ill is frightening, and undermined my own feelings of being able to trust myself.

On another occasion, after coming out of hospital I went into the surgery and was certain that my partners wanted me to leave the practice. I had no evidence, but felt unable to trust their reassurances. Eventually my wife spoke to the practice manager and she tried to reassure me it was OK. I was inclined to not even trust my wife until I gained enough insight to think that this was getting ridiculous, my wife had nothing to gain from this. I realised I was having paranoid-style beliefs which I could see, at least in part, were not true. I had no trouble then believing my wife, but never completely felt comfortable with all my partners. This had two effects. Firstly, and most obviously, it undermined relationships within the practice. How do you maintain professional relationships when you feel you can't trust colleagues and realise that this is related to your own inability to trust? How can they work with you when you feel you don't trust them, but have no reason to feel that way? The second effect is more internal. I realised that my own internal world was distorted. My very thinking was flawed, but exactly to what extent and in what ways I could not see because I was inside my own thoughts. I found it hard to find any reference points on which to make judgements. Clinical work can fairly easily be checked out, but what of relationships? Was I being a nasty suspicious person, rejecting the help my friends could offer, or was I the victim of an undiscovered plot? In the end I depended on the advice and reality checking of a small number of close friends and professionals, but my own confidence plummeted.

Bizarre stuff with no insight

Complete loss of insight can be a less difficult experience than partial insight. One member of our group describes a manic episode where she was completely taken over by delusional thinking. This she describes as being a relief from the pains of her illness. For me the only time I lost complete insight was still painful. Sitting in the GP co-op one evening I was struck suddenly first that a curtain rail was going to trap and hang me, and then that the wires at the back of the computer were coming to strangle me. Scary stuff, and very real for a few moments until things returned to normal and I was left worrying that this was a pretty bizarre experience and I was losing it. Perhaps I had not completely lost insight after all if I could so quickly see how bizarre it was.

When being admitted to hospital for the first time, I was asked what I was thinking when I first entered my room. 'Just checking the room out for suicide potential, as you do with a hotel room etc.' For some reason they put me on one-to-one observation straight away. I felt frustrated that my carers overreacted and took away any possible suicide hazard. I simply could not understand what was happening and why and felt bemused and powerless. Simple reason could no longer inform me of reality, but instead locked me in a false world disconnected from those around me. It took months for me to let go of that belief, slowly gaining partial insight and as a result feeling my sense of security in my own judgement become gradually undermined and then more gradually rebuilt. I still from time to time wonder if my thinking had been really so bizarre in the circumstances. Perhaps I was right, that people do check out hotel rooms for suicide potential. Was I so out of touch with normality, or am I even now, five years on, still a bit screwed up and think in odd ways? I suspect the truth is somewhere inbetween. I guess the scars of past bizarre thinking live on in the undermined judgement that remains.

Self-harm

Self-harm is a well known phenomenon. All those people turning up in A&E with minor cuts to suture and dress and young people taking smallish overdoses. These are the stereotypes, and bring with them feelings of manipulation, acting out feelings in a public and inappropriate way, leading to professionals feeling negative and unempathic. We, as professionals, feel angry and manipulated, and indeed patients will often agree that their behaviour is designed to effect change in others. This seems particularly so with overdoses. Like all stereotypes, there is some truth in this, but the stories of DSN members revealed in this book bring out a different picture, a far more complex picture, of perhaps a different type of self-harm.

First, self-harm comes in very many forms. Some people go in for cutting, with scalpels, scissors and knives, others for burning with liquid nitrogen, and yet others for eating problems, either bingeing, vomiting or purging. As doctors we have access to a wide range of potentially hazardous instruments and substances, and in my practice my partner and practice nurse try to ensure that I have limited access to scalpel blades and scissors, and the liquid nitrogen store key is kept by the practice manager and partner to try to limit the self-harm opportunities. It helps, but doesn't completely stop it.

Of course, as doctors we also know what is truly dangerous and what will just be enough to achieve what we feel we need from self-harming. So what are we trying to achieve? It seems there are two main motives for self-harming: release and punishment.

The main reason is relief from overwhelming feelings. So often people say that they vomit, cut etc. as a way of dealing with feelings they otherwise would not be able to cope with. Obviously this is a maladaptive response, but it does make reasonable sense. Imagine being in a small group education meeting and suddenly something happens that triggers feelings of panic, humiliation, hatred of oneself and extreme vulnerability. Then a quick trip to the loo to vomit, to clear those impossible feelings, makes sense. Equally when the feelings include a strong sense of self-hatred a quick cut to draw blood and release a shot of adrenalin can stop it before it turns to more lethal ways of harming. Interestingly in other literature overdose tends not to be used in this way. This is presumably because, unlike cutting and vomiting, there is no immediate affect from overdose.

The second main reason for self-harming is simple self-hatred, a desire to punish oneself for being who you are. One person describes cutting etc. deliberately to cause scars that will last, and to cause pain, to show to himself and to the world what a worthless person he is. However, with this degree of anger turned in into self-destructive behaviour there is a significant risk of loss of control which can lead on to clearly more lethal behaviours.

Perhaps the most obvious thing about doctors self-harming, and a lot of other individuals too, is the secrecy. Unlike the stereotype, the people in our group hardly ever present to health professionals with self-harming. OK, so we can treat minor injuries ourselves, and we can be very skilled at managing our eating behaviours. But we hide our wounds, and remain silent about our vomiting. Cutting on the arms may be hidden with long sleeves, but wounds on the top of the leg or abdomen can be hidden without the sometimes self-conscious need to wear long sleeves. I have got to the stage where I will admit to close friends and professionals when asked, a few days after the event, but the offer to speak to a trusted friend before I self-harm is too hard to take up. The problem is shame. We are grown-ups and not supposed to do this. The behaviour is disgusting and for those who bear scars, they too are disgusting, and by extension we as people must be disgusting.

One person's experience of self-harm behaviours

I started self-harming when I was nine years old, hitting myself with a hammer. I was sulking in the shed and discovered accidentally if I hurt myself I felt better. When I was 13 I started cutting myself with my razor for similar reasons. It was only very superficial and I had no real depressive symptoms at the time. When I was 18 I began to feel very sad all the time and thoughts of hanging became increasingly intrusive. The cutting became more and more frequent, with serious damage, and I still felt very low. I cut to *stop* me killing myself, as by the time I had done it, gone to A&E, and got stitched, the thoughts were again manageable.

I had similar thoughts with my anorexia/bulimia. It kept thoughts of suicide at bay. It started when I was 15 and when I was at university I spent £50 a day on food. I used to get an adrenalin rush from thinking where I would get the money – begging my bank manager, stealing food from both shops and flatmates. I would eat it then throw up until I shook and could barely walk. Then I would repeat the cycle again and again, often staying up all night.

When I was 20 I realised I had to stop as I couldn't do wards while I had huge cuts on my arm. So I arranged an admission with my CPN and was in over my 21st birthday. I stopped the day before my birthday and haven't done it since.

About two years later I did the same with my eating and to help they put me on 60mg of Prozac, which is supposed to reduce bingeing. I felt really well and a week later I met my husband, stopped the Prozac, and remained well for two years. However, recently I was readmitted and was sectioned. Prior to admission and while sectioned, I started bulimia again, but this improved when I became well and is now totally gone.

I think I used the adrenalin and other brain chemicals from these activities as an antidepressant but I think there are many reasons people do this.

I think a lot of my problems improved as the depression resolved, but both of these problems are addictive and, as with other forms of dependence, will only improve if you want them to.

I have developed alternatives to cutting that are less severe, such as swapping from cutting to waxing my arms, or drawing red lines on my arms. There is also a role for displacement activity, and having someone available twenty-four hours a day to talk to when you feel like cutting.

Eating disorders, in particular anorexia, really need specialist treatment with food diaries, dietician input and often counselling or psychotherapy.

Fiona Donnolly

So, what conclusions can we come to on this?

First, put aside any preconceived ideas about self-harm. Each person in our group with self-harm behaviour is different and unique, and none of them fit the popular A&E stereotype.

In particular, the motivation of eating disorders is complex and varies from person to person. Fiona clearly describes an adrenalin rush from her bulimia behaviour, which I recognise from my cutting behaviour. (Liquid nitrogen burns take a day or two to show and so there is no rush, and so will not relieve any acute feelings. They are, however, good at scarring and so are more helpful when self-hatred demands that it leaves its mark.) However, another group member with bulimia gets no adrenalin rush and minimises the effects of the vomiting by taking potassium supplements. As always, the key is to listen to individual stories.

Second, remember that the secrecy speaks of extreme shame, so the issue needs to be discussed with care. In writing my bits of this book I have tried to be as open as possible about my illness, and I try to live my life being upfront about it, but this little section on self-harm is particularly difficult. I have shied away from being as open as I could have been, such is the power of shame. Handle with care.

Finally, given that self-harm is usually a way of relieving intolerable feelings, don't expect us to stop easily. It may be possible to reduce the activity fairly dramatically through reducing risk opportunities and focusing on the behaviour itself, but in the end it will only be by dealing with the underlying issues that lead to the intolerable feelings that it will be possible to drop it completely.

Summary

- Normal defences occur in the mentally ill as well as the well.
- Mental illness leads to a distancing from reality which can become quite extreme.
- When you lose insight you really can't understand another person's reactions and thinking. This can be confusing and frightening.
- Self-harm is not uncommon, but often hidden and associated with extreme shame.
- Self-harm is a way of relieving tension and intolerable feelings quickly.
- Self-harm is a way of punishing oneself and hating oneself.
- In our group self-harm is not seen as a way of effecting change in others.

Chapter 18

Key issues for medical students and schools

Anon

Disabled students and doctors, including those with mental health problems, can have a very positive impact on the medical profession. This diversity would more accurately reflect the patient population, help to break down old, paternalistic attitudes and challenge stigma. This is important within the medical profession, as evidence suggests that stigma is widespread.[1] A more accepting and accessible culture would help the medical profession to address its own problems more effectively, as it is well known that there are increased rates of mental health problems and clinically significant psychological distress in doctors compared with the general population[2,3] and evidence that this is also true for medical students.[4–6] The main problems include affective disorders[7] and substance use disorders.[8,9] Eating disorders seem to be a problem anecdotally but there is little evidence to back this up.[10] This chapter will discuss issues which often concern students and highlight recent changes in the law which provide a framework for protecting students' rights, making this an exciting time for change in medical education.

Far from blanket positive or negative discrimination, all students should be treated fairly on the basis of their individual cases and should be helped and supported as much as possible in fulfilling their potential without compromising current or future patient care. This is not always easy, as the medical course provides some unique challenges and barriers to help-seeking behaviour such as fitness to practise issues, so it is important that services provided are tailored to the needs of students and do not shy away from important issues. However, this is still a very rewarding and important field since it allows us to influence the future of the profession. It has been shown that students mimic the attitudes of their teachers and the process of professionalisation starts early.[11]

Disability Discrimination Act 1995 (DDA)

I have used the word 'disabled' deliberately, as many people with mental health problems will be covered by the DDA's definition of disability. The DDA has recently been amended to include education by the Special Educational Needs and Disability Act 2001 (SENDA), which came into force in 2002 as Part IV of the DDA. This law is still recent, meaning that there is very little case law to clarify the precise meanings of some of these terms and its practical application.

Definition of disability

Under the Act, the effect of a disability must be substantial, long-term and adverse and affect a person's abilities to carry out normal day-to-day activities.[12] These definitions relate to untreated state functioning and a person is still covered by the Act once they have recovered.

Discrimination

The Act defines discrimination by the Responsible Body as occurring in two ways:[13,14]

- **Less favourable treatment** of the disabled person, for reasons relating to the person's disability that cannot be **justified** (e.g. by **reasons that are material and substantial**).
- **Failure to make reasonable adjustments** that place or are likely to place disabled applicants, students or potential students at a **substantial disadvantage** compared to their non-disabled peers. A substantial disadvantage is one that entails time, inconvenience, effort or discomfort compared to other people or students and which is more than minor or trivial.

Who is covered?

The scope of the Act is very broad and includes applicants and potential students, full-, part-time and visiting students.

Reasonable adjustments

The Act does not define what reasonable adjustments may be. What is 'reasonable' varies according to circumstances: it will be affected by the need to maintain academic standards, the nature of the institution, its size and resources, the effect of the disability on the individual and other factors. Skill, the UK charity for students with disabilities, has given examples for students with mental health problems:[15]

- extra support and help with planning before or during exam and assessment periods
- exam officers to be aware that problems may arise during exam periods
- support from welfare and counselling staff
- a named contact to go to for support when necessary
- flexibility in attendance and punctuality if treatments or therapies are tightly scheduled or during times when difficulties are worse than usual
- computer equipment to enable you to study at home
- a quiet room to rest in
- contact from staff during any periods of time away from studies

- maintenance of confidentiality about your mental health difficulties
- sufficient information and awareness amongst staff who do know about your difficulties to prevent major misconceptions.

I have found that at their worst medical schools can be quite inflexible and sometimes dogmatic when considering adjustments, presumably because this is a recent development and the course itself is highly structured and must fulfil GMC requirements, e.g. the undergraduate curriculum must usually be completed in seven years, excluding intercalated degrees.[16] In fact, as representatives from Skill would point out, adjustments can be wide-ranging provided that there is a clear idea of the key competencies actually being tested,[17] i.e. particular knowledge rather than the stamina to sit a three hour exam. University procedures may be rigid in themselves and care should be taken to avoid invoking disciplinary procedures too arbitrarily or inappropriately against a student with mental health problems at the institution.[18] There should not be a punitive approach. If invoked, the format of these procedures should not exacerbate the student's health problem.

Responsible bodies

Despite its repeated assertions that it has 'no direct statutory role in matters of student health and conduct',[19] the GMC (General Medical Council) is classed as a responsible body for making adjustments under the DDA. For most higher education courses, the responsible body is the university. In medicine it is a combination of the university and GMC. The GMC accredits the course and examinations and to this extent, universities are *responsible* for making adaptations and the GMC for deciding *whether* adaptations will be made.[14] Further legislation is in progress to clarify the duties of responsible bodies. Admittedly, the GMC's track record with disability, particularly Heidi Cox's case, leaves something to be desired.[20]

Disclosure

Under the DDA, the responsible body must know or could have reasonably known about an individual's disability for discrimination to take place. The relevant code of practice brings out some important points:[14]

- The institution's culture and atmosphere must facilitate disclosure, e.g. to be open and welcoming to disability.
- The responsible body must have taken reasonable steps to find out about the disability and be proactive in encouraging people to disclose disabilities. This may include publicising services and adaptations, and providing opportunities for students to tell staff in confidence.
- Once the student has disclosed to one person, the responsible body may not be able to claim that it did not know, unless the student asks for it to be kept confidential. (This is sensitive personal data and should be dealt with according to the institution's confidentiality policy and the Data Protection Act 1998 in any case.)

- Responsible bodies have an anticipatory duty to plan what adaptations may be needed, so that they may not be able to claim lack of notice as a defence.

Resolving disputes

Problems can be resolved either formally or informally within the university, through its own procedures, through mediation (the DRC has set up the Disability Conciliation Service which provides rights-focused mediation for disputes under the Act) or in a court of law.[13] Using internal procedures is often preferable because this can be much quicker, less confrontational, requires less time to prepare and has none of the emotional and financial cost sometimes associated with court cases. Also, the solutions that a court can provide may be quite limited, e.g. financial compensation and another type of action, judicial review, may be required to challenge university decisions if the institution may have failed to follow its own procedures.

Tips on resolving disputes

- **Kill the monster while it's small!** Do something early before the consequences get too big.
- **Find someone to talk to** that you trust, as this can be a difficult time and another opinion will help you to be objective – you really need to be.
- **Get everything in writing** as recall can be very subjective.
- **Know what you want, what your rights are and communicate clearly** – don't assume that people know certain facts or be too afraid to speak up because of differences in status.
- **Don't make it personal** – don't take others' actions personally, however hurtful, and always be professional when interacting with people. It can be helpful to give people a way to back down gracefully, i.e. pointing out an action which is in line with their own policies, rather than being too accusatory or humiliating.
- **Keep knocking on doors!** You can't always predict who'll help you and need to avoid being disadvantaged by individual differences. Using other university services as a sort of ambassador or intermediary can be very helpful. Examples include university disability officers, senior tutors, specialist mental health officers or welfare services.
- **Seek outside advice early** – again, this helps you to stay objective and be better informed. Examples include Skill (the UK charity for students with disabilities), DRC, NUS education unit, BMA medical students committee or BMA industrial relations officers.

Other legislation

Common law

Universities owe their students a duty of care, which means that services should be provided with 'reasonable care and skill'. This duty of care may be enhanced for vulnerable students. A recent report by AMOSSHE (Association of Managers of Student Services in Higher Education) has identified some principles of good practice for student support services and these could easily be applied to other areas. They include effective provision of services and liaison with the student body; transparency, honesty and designated responsibility; clear policies and procedures; and training, staff development and support.[21]

Human Rights Act 1998

The Human Rights Act is wide-ranging and includes the right to education (First Protocol, Article 2) and prohibition of discrimination (Article 14), although disability is not explicitly stated.[22] It is possible that this, particularly Article 2 of the First Protocol, will apply to higher education, and a recent report by Eversheds solicitors suggests that universities should proceed as if it did apply.[23]

Applications and admission

In an ideal world students would identify their needs as early as possible so that suitable adjustments could be made for them. In the real world, few applicants declare a disability on their UCAS forms; in the 2001/02 application cycle 0.82% of applicants declared a disability, and a tiny fraction of these declared a mental health problem. Compared with this, HESA statistics show that 4.1% of students with a disability registered on higher education courses in the 2000/01 academic year.[24] There may be a number of reasons for this, including lack of knowledge about the scope of 'disability' and fear of stigma.[25] It isn't helped by this section being on the front of the first page and not confidential from the rest of the application as occupational health forms for employment normally are.

When I applied, potential applicants with any significant mental or physical impairment were strongly discouraged by some parties. I remember one speaker saying this at a conference I attended and it being mentioned in an institution's application material. This hampered my seeking help and disclosing what was happening when I became ill. Information available to potential applicants has changed a lot and in general universities are much more aware of disability issues. However, research shows that students still have similar perceived norms,[26] so any positive, inclusive messages about mental health cannot be overstated at any time. In general, medical school websites make very little reference to mental health, let alone anything positive.[27]

'Selectionism' and fitness to enter

I have occasionally come across attitudes which view mental illness as a total bar to practising medicine or a result of failures in selecting the right students. It is true that practising medicine may not be possible for some applicants with disabilities or health problems, but both viewpoints are extremely flawed. First, they cover a very diverse area, where conditions have a wide range of severities and impact on people's lives. They penalise people for seeking help; we are all aware of the illness iceberg and demographic variations in seeking help. They foster a culture of denial; people in denial and unaware of their own limitations or unable to admit to them may be more dangerous. They also fail to take into account the prevalence of mental illness and age of onset of common conditions. A popular statistic is that 1 in 4 of us will be experiencing mental distress at any one time,[28] and 1 in 6 will be experiencing significant mental health problems.[29] This potentially rules out a large group of applicants, possibly according to prejudice and misconception. The age of onset of many adult psychiatric disorders is around the age of majority or later,[30] so this form of selection may highlight candidates who have a history of childhood or adolescent disorders that may not persist, but be ineffective in weeding out adult psychiatric disorders, as the majority of entrants are still in their late teens or early twenties. Perhaps recent proposals to include psychometric or personality testing to select applicants with certain personality traits stem from a similar viewpoint. In my view, mental illness is simply too prevalent and medical training and practice itself too great a risk factor for it ever to be selected out in this way, not to mention the problems created by selecting a particular 'type' of person for a very diverse profession. These attitudes also create significant barriers to seeking help. It seems ironic that the medical profession is well placed to lead the way in combating stigma yet a recent report claims that stigma towards employees' mental health problems is worse in the NHS than in the private sector.[31]

Many medical schools are now phasing in 'fitness to enter' schemes that assess the health status of applicants.[27] In an ideal world these may well be positive, illustrating the institution's awareness of disability and providing the opportunity to plan in advance. However, in the real world these need to be analysed very carefully. The measure can be seen as a positive step provided that it is used with care and skill, not as a means to discriminate. Unlike the UCAS form, where there is no penalty for non-disclosure, fitness to enter schemes may incorporate such a penalty. Take an example from Nottingham's website: 'Failure to disclose information which directly relates to your fitness to practise will result in the termination of your medical school course'.[32] So it is vital that a culture which genuinely facilitates disclosure is created, and it is questionable how it is possible to do this on paper before the applicant is enrolled.

Disclosure

Knowing what and when to disclose can seem particularly frightening and perilous. I remember that I could hardly speak when I first had to disclose to a member of my faculty (this isn't like me), as I was so frightened of being chucked out or ruining my career. Sometimes this can be made worse by the blurring of professional boundaries – the doctors teaching you don't or shouldn't need to be involved in your clinical care! It can be helpful to remember a concept from Occupational Health, that disclosure to line managers (e.g. those who directly supervise and assess you) should be avoided where possible as it can harm their objectivity. However, this can be helpful in some circumstances. Disclosure will always be a difficult issue and the only advice I can give is to trust your instincts and remember that information can't be un-disclosed. The majority of staff who

I've told about my illness have been positive, some surprisingly so, but I've found this very hard to predict.

Seeking help

My experiences, anecdotal evidence and research all point to barriers to seeking help. Some of the most frequently cited are concerns about confidentiality, impact on future career and academic impartiality.[26] These are linked to perceived norms stating that experiencing a mental health problem may be viewed as a weakness that has negative implications on subsequent career progression.[26] There is often a conflict between these needs and perceptions and the services provided. For instance, medical school staff, e.g. clinical tutors, are often suggested as the first point of contact, which isn't compatible with this viewpoint. Students have also been shown to have little knowledge of the services available. These barriers must be broken down. A culture needs to be created where seeking help for a mental health problem is seen as a positive step and a good reason to seek help early[33] and experiencing mental health problems isn't a sign of weakness or ruinous to a career.

Student support

In general, experiencing mental health problems can be isolating, demoralising and disempowering. Support should be provided in ways which challenge this, much as Christopher Spence aimed to counteract similar effects of HIV when setting up the London Lighthouse.[34] Staff often need to remember that their students are adults with rights and autonomy. Involving students in decision making and service provision is actually very important, both from a rights-based and an empowerment perspective. It's not acceptable that assumptions are made about disease states or what students need and that decisions are made behind closed doors without full accountability or transparency. Students should be involved at an individual and university-wide level in determining service provision wherever possible.

Many systems exist to provide emotional and practical help to students while at university. Examples include:

- friends and family
- personal tutors
- other university staff e.g. porters or cleaners if in halls
- careers service
- disability service
- counselling service
- health centre
- chaplaincy
- welfare service
- NUS
- specialist mental health officers.

Students with mental health problems will have access to all the same services as their healthy counterparts but these services should have adequate training/resources to adapt to meet their needs, e.g. careers talking about issues of disclosure, and should be accessible. Mentally ill medical students are almost doubly isolated from these services because medical schools tend to be set apart from universities. This isn't necessarily geographical, but students often have different term dates, workloads or are away on clinical placements. In my own experience I have noticed a culture of separateness where the medical school seems to be a self-contained unit different from the rest of the university. This has wider resonance, as sometimes medical schools appear to act autonomously, disregarding university-wide policies. Students studying other subjects may receive more publicity about adaptations, be provided with personal tutors etc., but not necessarily medical students. I've also noticed attitudes which suggest that medical students don't need such forms of support, that they should be robust enough to address the challenges of the course and university life without such measures. More worrying is the culture created and the future impact on students. Research suggests that attitudes and help-seeking behaviours are formed early and that training and pre-training influences are likely to play a role in the profession's excess morbidity and mortality from mental health related causes.[26] Until medicine can stamp out these views it will never create a culture which is truly open and inclusive to disability, particularly mental illness, and will hamper its members from seeking help. Hardly something that a profession with mortality statistics like medicine[2] should be striving for.

Services and support must be provided in line with students' needs, and not based on assumptions, and stigma must be addressed.

A range of central and departmental services should be provided so that students have the option of seeking help outside their department and factors giving rise to inequalities in provision, i.e. hours and location, must be addressed and solved creatively. Personal tutors often play a key role in being one of the first points of contact for students, with numbers accessing them for help being second highest after friends and family.[35] If appropriately trained, they are well placed to refer students to other, more specialist services. Barriers to seeking help in medical education may mean that this system doesn't work as well. In that case, confidentiality guidelines and the independence of personal tutors needs to be emphasised. Similar support could also be provided in a number of other ways, for instance mentoring by junior doctors or GPs. Provisions could include adequately trained and motivated personal tutors who are only responsible for welfare and are outside the student's working/assessment group. Clear, publicised policies on confidentiality and record keeping and regular consultations with students are vital, as are appealing ways of getting their attention when publicising services.

Health education for healthcare students

An interesting conclusion of the Royal College of Psychiatrists' report into the mental health of students is that healthcare students should have teaching about their own wellbeing. For instance, to explain the risks and promote more positive norms and '. . . a culture of self-awareness in which the students' own experience can be disclosed and discussed as part of a reflective learning paradigm'.[33] This would be an ideal situation; the student should not feel under pressure to disclose, however.

Staff attitudes

A 'good attitude' can probably be defined as one that is non-judgemental and accepting, that values the unique contribution that mental health service users can make in medicine without letting go of objectivity or wider responsibilities. It is ideally backed up by knowledge and experience of mental health issues. During my training I've encountered a wide range of attitudes to mental illness from the overwhelmingly positive and occasionally unrealistic through to ignorance, paternalism, people being unsure of how to treat me, making assumptions and the occasional mild form of prejudice. These have been directed both towards mental illness in general and towards individuals, including myself. It can be quite uncomfortable when someone is being negative about mentally ill people without realising that you are one. Many responses have been positive and some come from some surprising sources, but it has been almost impossible to predict how people will react. This is one reason why my first attempts at disclosure were so terrifying. In general I have been treated well while at medical school; I have occasionally been discriminated against and I believe that this was more the result of ignorance and lack of training than anything else. It has been suggested to me that the increased emphasis on political correctness hampers people when dealing with mentally ill students but I'm really not sure about this.

Fitness to practise

Research suggests that the majority of medical academics find it more challenging to deal with students who have mental health problems rather than other disabilities. This is especially true in the area of fitness to practise where decisions are particularly agonising and involve matching current and predicted future health to the individual's ability to complete the tasks required of them.[36] This highlights the fact that decisions on fitness to practise are never easy but are made worse by the lack of resources and guidance available. The GMC *Guidance on Student Health and Conduct* states that:

> Subject to meeting a University's regulations, anyone can graduate provided that they meet all the outcomes and curriculum require-ments in *Tomorrow's Doctors*. The view of the GMC is that students with a wide range of disabilities or health conditions can achieve the prescribed standards of knowledge, skills, attitudes and behaviour.[19]

One major problem seems to be a lack of uniformity between institutions and possible interpretations of policies and guidance, which can vary widely because guidelines aren't that specific. For instance, the information provided on medical school websites about student health, disability and fitness to practise policies varies widely.[27,36] The outcomes mentioned above and listed in other documents like the *QAA Subject Benchmarks for Medicine* need to be elaborated on so that there is a detailed, national list of competencies expected of new medical graduates and required for students to learn on the course, as suggested by the DIVERSE project[27] and Skill Scotland.[36] This would decrease the wide range of interpretations available. Also, disability professionals should be involved in determining fitness to enter and practise; this has been widely recommended.[27] This could include Disability Officers, Occupational Health doctors and other relevant specialists. However, stigma in the NHS must be tackled in order to avoid the potential for these processes being discriminatory. Disabled doctors have an important role to play in developing fitness to enter and practise procedures and guidelines, as they will have one of the most accurate perspectives of the impact of illness on the practice of medicine.

Transition to work

The medical degree is vocational and really a preparation for starting work as a doctor. Junior doctors obviously work longer hours and have more responsibility than medical students; these are all potential sources of stress and may have serious consequences. Hence the transition to work needs to be managed carefully. Graduates or students may need input and support from a variety of areas including postgraduate deaneries, Occupational Health, careers advice, informal support and mentoring, and good primary and secondary care. Postgraduate training is potentially more flexible than undergraduate training; for instance, it is now possible to train part-time as a postgraduate including the pre-registration year.[16] In order to make these adjustments, deaneries need to be provided with information but this should be with the students' consent and co-operation unless they are perceived to be a public danger. Obviously, information about an individual's health status should not be included in employment references.

A good occupational health service could be important in helping an individual start their working life and ideally, because medicine is such a vocational course, this support would be available during the degree, particularly in the clinical years. It's unfortunate that evidence suggests that the NHS occupational health service provision is patchy and does not offer specialist psychiatric advice with very few exceptions, despite evidence suggesting that 50% of those attending may have psychological or psychiatric problems.[1] Provision may be even more patchy at universities with an estimate of 50% being covered.[27] Careers advice may also be useful around this time. Ideally it needs to be doubly specialist and able to give specific information about medical careers and issues around disability. This may be difficult to find, as medical schools may have little provision of careers advice for any student. There is some provision in the private sector.

The medical culture itself may be unwelcoming, I remember an off the cuff comment from a Royal College careers day speaker referring to gaps in someone's CV: '. . . they'll think you were mad or something . . .'. The report of the Daksha Emson Inquiry indicated that the NHS may be far worse at stigmatising mental health in its employees compared to the private sector.[1] Added to mistrust about NHS confidentiality, this makes for a difficult situation. However, it is not an impossible one, as there are many signs of positive change and many people working in the NHS who don't discriminate against their colleagues. Also, medical students and graduates are highly able and resourceful, given the stringent entrance requirements, so are more likely than most to overcome these problems and change the current situation for the better. The current situation is hardly static, as this is a significant time of change for people with all disabilities in medicine.

Conclusion

The law against discrimination should really be taken as a bare minimum, as suggested by the DRC in its Code of Practice. Adhering to the letter of the law just to avoid prosecution can't really take the place of the institution-wide positive attitude to students with disabilities, including mental health problems, that is so vital. It also doesn't encourage any innovation above and beyond these quite modest requirements. I hope it is clear that these recent changes do not advocate the rights of the student over and above the rights of the general public, whom they'll eventually serve, but give rise to a more balanced approach where students have more rights where they once had very few.

I have tried to give as much of a neutral, unbiased view as possible when writing this. Undoubtedly I have failed in some areas simply because I've been swayed by certain experiences, so I'm sorry for sounding excessively negative in some areas. I think it is important to emphasise that the future isn't an excessively bleak one. Change in the areas I've described is happening fast, so the overall message should be one of hope for the future. Chapter 28 gives details of organisations that may be helpful if you are a medical student experiencing difficulties.

References

1 North East London Strategic Health Authority (2003) *Report of an independent inquiry into the care and treatment of Daksha Emson MBBS, MRCPsych, MSc and her daughter Freya.* North East London Strategic Health Authority, London.
2 Office of Population Censuses and Surveys (1995) *Occupational Health Decennial Supplement for England and Wales.* HMSO, London.
3 Firth-Cozens J (1989) Stress in medical undergraduates and house officers. *Br J Hosp Med.* **41(2)**: 161–4.
4 Roberts LW, Warner TD and Trumpower D (2000) Caring for medical students as patients: access to services and care-seeking practices of 1027 students at non-medical schools. Collaborative Research Group on Medical Student Healthcare. *Acad Med.* **75(3)**: 272–7.
5 Okasha A, Lotaif F and Sadek A (1981) Prevalence of suicidal feelings in a sample of non-consulting medical students. *Acta Psychiatr Scand.* **63(5)**: 409–15.
6 Chan DW (1991) Depressive symptoms and depressed mood among Chinese medical students in Hong Kong. *Compr Psychiatry.* **32(2)**: 170–80.
7 Steker T (2004) Well-being in an academic environment. *Med Educ.* **38(5)**: 465–78.
8 Baldwin DC, Hughes PH, Conrad SE, Storr CL and Sheehan DV (1991) Substance use among senior medical students: a survey of 23 medical schools. *JAMA.* **265**: 2074–8.

9 Newbury-Birch D, Walshaw D and Kamali F (2001) Drink and drugs: from medical students to doctors. *Drug Alcohol Depend.* **64(3)**: 265–70.

10 Szweda S and Thorne P (2002) The prevalence of eating disorders in female health care students. *Occup Med (Lond).* **52(3)**: 113–19.

11 Sinclair S (1997) *Making Doctors.* Berg, Oxford.

12 HMSO The Disability Discrimination Act (1995). *Guidance on Matters to be Taken into Account in Determining Questions Relating to the Definition of Disability.* HMSO, London.

13 *Disability Discrimination Act 1995.* HMSO, London.

14 DRC (2002) *Code of Practice for Providers of Post-16 Education and Related Services.* DRC, London.

15 Skill (2004) *The Needs of Students in Further and Higher Education.* Skill, London.

16 GMC (2003) *Tomorrow's Doctors.* GMC, London.

17 Skill (2002) *The Disability Discrimination Act Part 4: Examinations and assessment good practice guide.* Skill, London.

18 CVCP (now Universities UK) (2000) *Guidelines on Student Mental Health Policies and Procedures for Higher Education.* CVCP, London.

19 GMC (2002) *Guidance on Student Health and Conduct.* GMC, London.

20 Taysum P (2002) The GMC has set a precedent for discriminating against disabled medical students. *BMJ.* **324**: S199.

21 AMOSSHE. *Responding to Student Mental Health Issues; 'duty of care' responsibilities for student services in higher education.* AMOSSHE, Birmingham.

22 *Human Rights Act 1998.* HMSO, London.

23 Eversheds Solicitors (2001) *Fitness to Practise in the Medical Profession – A report to Universities UK and the Council of Heads of Medical Schools by Eversheds Solicitors.* Eversheds, London.

24 DEMOS project. Online Materials for staff disability awareness [online] updated February 2003 [cited August 2004] Admissions of disabled applicants to Higher Education (HE). Available at: http://jarmin.com/demos/course/admiss/index.html.

25 Student Mental Health (Lancaster University) (2002) *Planning, Guidance and Training Manual.* www.studentmentalhealth.org.uk/index.htm.

26 Chew-Graham CA, Rogers A and Yassin N (2003) 'I wouldn't want it on my CV or their records': medical students' experiences of help-seeking for mental health problems. *Medical Education.* **37**: 83.

27 Tynan A (2004) *The Sequel to Pushing the Boat Out.* LTSN01 special report 3. Newcastle-upon-Tyne.

28 Goldberg D and Huxley P (1982) *Common Mental Disorders.* Routledge, London.

29 ONS (2000) *Psychiatric Morbidity Among Adults Living in Private Households in Great Britain.* ONS, London.

30 Gelder M, Lopez-Ibor J and Andreasen N (eds) (2000) *New Oxford Textbook of Psychiatry.* OUP, Oxford.

31 North East London Strategic Health Authority (2003) *Report of an independent inquiry into the care and treatment of Daksha Emson MBBS, MRCPsych, MSc and her daughter Freya.* North East London Strategic Health Authority, London.

32 Nottingham University. Applying for Medicine [online] Available at: http://www.nottingham.ac.uk/mhs/admissions/applying.html#disab.

33 Royal College of Psychiatrists (2003) *The Mental Health of Students in Higher Education.* RCPsych, London.

34 Spence C (1996) *On Watch: Views from the Lighthouse.* Continuum, London.

35 Grant A (2002) Identifying and responding to students' concerns: a whole institutional approach. In: N Stanley and J Manthorpe (eds) *Students' Mental Health Needs: problems and responses.* Jessica Kingsley Publishers, London.

36 Tynan A. *Pushing the Boat Out.* LTSN-0I. Newcastle-upon-Tyne.

Chapter 19

Being a doctor with an illness to patients with an illness

Helen Cox, Petre Jones and Anon

In this chapter Helen Cox, a Psychiatry SpR from Yorkshire, Petre Jones, a GP from inner city Newham in East London, and Anon, another GP, look at their illnesses and how they have altered the way they practise medicine. Each suffers from an affective disorder, and each continues to work in clinical practice.

Physician heal thyself?

I was in my fourth psychiatric SHO job when I became depressed. My work had given me an understanding of emotional distress and the beliefs that normal feelings should not be psychiatrised and that if you play the game and comply, mental illness does not have to rule your life. My illness gave me a much more real appreciation of the symptoms we treat. Since returning to work 18 months ago I have become section 12 approved, passed part 2 and been offered an SpR post which I will start shortly.

When I returned to work after having been severely depressed I had a much deeper and broader understanding of the experience of mental illness, although I recognise that illness affects each person differently, and I would never assume that patients experience their symptoms in the same way I did mine.

I now appreciate how 'bodily' and physical a depressive illness can feel. For me it was a heavy empty exhausted dragging feeling which was worse than the sadness, and knowing this it is little wonder that so many depressed patients present to other branches of medicine with a conviction that they are 'physically' ill.

I recall having great difficulty thinking and coping with day-to-day tasks, particularly the post, and since returning to work I have been more aware of helping patients to access benefits advice etc., as simple forms feel insurmountable at times. I also pass on advice I received about reading children's novels, as the sentences are shorter and the plots simpler for befuddled brains to cope with.

While unwell I made some poor decisions and got my finances into a terrible mess. My illness had far-reaching effects on my life. This has affected my view on detention under the Mental Health Act, as I do not think that being detained should be regarded as punitive but as an opportunity to get well. When I assess people under the Act I am more aware of the damage that can be done to someone's life and relationships by their illness. I bear in mind not only the disadvantages of being detained but also the disadvantages of being left to one's own devices with abnormal thoughts and behaviour.

I was resistant to treatment and had to try five antidepressants as well as antipsychotics, night sedation and lithium before effective combinations were found. I have therefore experienced a lot of drug side effects first hand. Even now I am struggling with enormous weight gain from the mirtazepine combined with lithium, and the hassle of three-monthly blood tests and obtaining monthly repeat prescriptions while working full-time. Patients often cite the weight gain or tiredness or funny taste in their mouth or the hassle as reasons for stopping their meds, and then they relapse. I think my own experience has made me less tolerant in this respect because in my opinion being tired, or the size of a house, is vastly preferable to incapacitating severe depression. Weight gain or lethargy will not kill you directly, but severe depression claims the lives of up to 15% of its victims. Patients seem to see the downside of medication or admission but forget to weigh up the benefits as well. In my case I have my life back, which is easily worth the side effects I experience.

During my episode I also had a very brief experience of elated mood and a period of psychosis. Both were actually a wonderful respite from the hideous feeling of the depression and I now have an appreciation of why manic patients do not want treating, and how psychosis serves a function in escaping an unbearable reality.

In summary, my illness has left me with a clearer understanding of the experience of psychiatric symptomatology and a stronger conviction that timely, effective treatment should be offered and accepted to relieve suffering and prevent damage to the patient and their life.

Helen Cox, Psychiatrist

Let it all hang out

Working as an inner city GP leaves you no real place to hide. Many of my patients know about my recurrent depression, and I'm sure many don't really care about it one way or the other. It was hard at first when patients asked me about my illness, but I don't want to hide it and I soon learned that for some it was about finding out about mental illness and perhaps destigmatising it (oh, the doc has depression sometimes, perhaps it is a real illness) and for others there was a feeling that I would empathise more with their distress if I showed myself also to be human. I now often use how they react to my illness as a contrast to how depressed people see themselves.

During my various stages of recovery I have had a number of treatments. As mentioned above, I too have been on a lot of tablets and so am confident using a wide range – perhaps more than the average GP. I did many hours of CBT, and the skills I learned, and the literature I acquired, I pass on to my patients and registrars. I even wrote a paper on CBT as a teaching tool. More importantly, though, my illness showed me and others round me that there is a huge gap in traditional services in inner city Newham, between the 'mild depression and anxiety disorders' and patients with 'severe enduring psychotic illness' who were often very damaged. In the middle were people like me, with severe illness, but not really dealt with by the local services. So, initially using PMS growth money (and 'expanding the envelope' of rules governing it), I led on setting up what has become the Newham Primary Care Consortium, which now has a Nurse Consultant, two other full-time CBT therapists, and a number of MSc psychology students, all based in local general practices.

I have also done some psychotherapy and have found myself applying some of the principles of this in my daily work.

I guess I went into medicine partly out of a desire to help, to 'make everything all better', and this in turn comes from needing to be seen as a 'good person' to counterbalance my internal reality of being useless and worthless. I am now conscious of being very keen to help people with mental health problems, but for different reasons, I think. Now it is more a thing about paying back for the help I have received in turning my life around, and also out of the simple fact of feeling confident dealing with these issues. I pick up depression more than my colleagues and more quickly in the consultation, which is something to do with transference and patients' minimal cues easily resonating with my own still raw issues. I don't see this as a problem, as on average GPs only pick up 50% of patients with depression, but there is obviously a danger of over-treatment and medicalising normal distress. With more complex people there is also a risk of allowing my own story to get tangled up with the patient's story, and in particular going away not being sure whether what I feel is my own reasonable distress or a resonating transference from the patient. I find it really important to talk to my colleague on a regular basis, with time away from the practice to run through difficult patients either of us have seen and acknowledge how we feel. I never did this before I was ill and felt the illness forced this upon me as a way to stay well, but it is really useful.

Mental Health Act sectioning is very difficult. In the past I would follow the letter of the law and try to apply it with as much compassion as I could. Now I find it a lot harder. I have never been sectioned, but have been in a situation where being sectioned could have cost me my job. I have also been in a situation in hospital where the treatment was so dreadful, and so divorced from what I expressed as my need, that I discharged myself, with the blessing of family and friends. My view on sectioning has hardened. When I assess people I ask myself 'Is this person's situation so bad, so perilous, that I can bring myself to inflict on them what is effectively detention without trial?' Sometimes it is, and like the surgeon in the battlefield operating without anaesthetic to save life, I will sign section papers, but often, with more community input and imagination, an informal route can be found.

As well as clinical general practice I do a lot of teaching. Part of our vocational training scheme involves running small case discussion groups looking at the emotional aspects of dealing with complex patients and complex situations. The group members know about my illness, but it is remarkable how often the group turns to the topic of doctor stress, suicide, 'personality disorder' and mental illness. I run the group with a co-leader so that when I am lost for words, and my mind freezes, she can keep things going. On many occasions it has fallen to my own registrar to rescue me in such situations. Supportive debriefings afterwards are vital.

Petre Jones

Things at work that are difficult for me

1 **Lack of sleep and/or food always makes my depression worse**. I become increasingly ratty when sleep-deprived, and feel my cognitive processes and decision-making abilities slowing down. Then the mood starts dipping, along with the negative thoughts – 'I'm no good as a doctor', 'I can't cope', 'I'll make a mistake' etc.

2 **Coping when people make comments about patients with a psychiatric diagnosis.** Do you 'come out' or keep quiet? It may feel like it's you personally they're insulting (a good example of personalisation, a common cognitive distortion), but even if not, relationships are likely to become strained. And if you 'come out' they may be too embarrassed to speak to you again, and so try to avoid you. But then, you're probably trying to avoid them as being unsympathetic . . .

3 **Coping with patients with the same problem as me.** I have depression, and so tend to identify with patients with depression. Sometimes this can result in over-involvement, at other times it can be difficult because their depression is not following the same pattern my own did. I don't think I deal with other psychiatric problems any better than anyone else.

4 **Coming out to patients, particularly when they say 'You don't know what it's like'.** I think that's certainly true for major depression; unless you've had it, you really can't grasp the full horrors of it. I work as a GP, and see quite a lot of patients with depression. I have 'come out' with a couple of them, but always in the past tense – 'I have had depression, and been on antidepressants' rather than the present 'I am still on antidepressants'. I feel I have a right to my own privacy and confidentiality, but on occasions, I have felt it right to disclose my history to certain patients. Usually I have been seeing them for some time, and they often suspect that I may have experienced depression from the inside, as I seem to know an awful lot about it. I don't feel it is helpful to say that I am still on antidepressants 10 years on; I am trying to encourage them that they will get better!

5 **Assessing suicidal intent.** As I have lived with spells of permanent suicidal ideas, but never acted on them, I find suicidal intent quite difficult to assess. Most people seem to think that thinking about suicide is a sign that you should be admitted at once. I found there were different levels to suicidal ideas, and that if you had *ever* thought seriously about suicide, then the ideas were likely to recur any time you were under pressure. Thinking about it in a general way, although distressing for the person concerned, does not worry me particularly as a doctor. Looking at everything around you and working out how you could use it to kill yourself seems to be the next step. Fixing on one particular method is a significant advance on the planning. I get concerned when someone has fixed on a method, and has then worked out how they will do it and arranged the means, e.g. bought the paracetamol and worked out when they will be alone to take it.

6 **Sectioning someone.** I find sectioning someone straightforward if they are a danger to someone else. That has usually been a fairly straightforward decision. However, I am very aware that when you section someone, you

take away all their rights, and add a significant episode to their medical history, which may have an impact on future employment and insurance issues. I find sectioning someone as a danger to themselves because they are depressed extremely difficult. A lot of this is because I am aware that depression does fluctuate, and so what I am seeing now may have improved in a few hours' time. The other problem is that I am now realising that my initial episode of depression as a medical student was not as mild as I had assumed at the time (after all, I managed to attend lectures most days). I now realise that if my flatmates had called a doctor to see me almost any evening, I would probably have been sectioned. For me, the bad spells tended to be in the evenings, and during these, I would hide in bed, crying and rocking, and have persistent thoughts of slitting my wrists with a scalpel (which I had). However, these episodes passed after some hours, and I was back to lectures the next day. So being aware of how I could fluctuate makes me very reluctant to section anybody with depression.

Anon, GP

Take-home thoughts

Each of these authors have a lot to say in common. They understand more about mental illness and its treatment, and pass on tips and skills that they learned when ill themselves. They are more empathic and aware of strong transferences and are keen to offer effective treatments to their patients and, in the case of Petre, set up a CBT service. Anon, however, describes clearly the tensions inherent in wanting to help, but also being vulnerable oneself. The personal experience gives new insight, but raises questions about how much to project these onto patients – the struggle between transference and classical counter-transference.

On the subject of sectioning they differ. Helen Cox's experience has led her to view detention under the MHA as a positive opportunity for the patient, whereas for Petre it is a sometime necessary evil. How much of this difference is due to experience of mental illness, and how much due to experience of primary care and secondary care? Anon's feelings about sectioning clearly derive from their experience of their own illness.

Summary

- Issue of how much to disclose to patients.
- Having been ill equips us with extra diagnostic and assessment skills in mental health.
- Transferences from patients can be strong. They can be useful but should be managed.
- Personal identification can lead to more motivation to treat.
- Mental Health Act assessments are a time of intense focus on these dilemmas.

Chapter 20

GMC Health Procedures and the sick doctor

Belinda Brewer

I am a part-time GP working and living in Chichester. I have a seven-year history of serious mental health problems. Fifteen months ago, following a serious suicide attempt, my GP and psychiatrist wrote to the General Medical Council for advice.

A month later I received a letter from the GMC, sent by special delivery, stating that the Health Screener believed my ability to practise might be seriously impaired by reason of Bipolar Affective Disorder. This was the start of the GMC's investigation into my fitness to practise under the Health Procedures.

This article explains the Health Procedures with respect to my own case and looks at alternatives. It is vital patients are protected from underperforming doctors at the same time as supporting doctors who perform well despite serious ill health.

Referral

The GMC receives information about a doctor's health from a range of sources, including concerned colleagues, the doctor's own GP or specialist, Occupational Health department and employers. Rarely, other professionals, e.g. the police or pharmacists, contact them.

Restrictions and recommendations

Once the GMC receive information regarding a doctor's health, the information is referred to one of three directorates: Health, Conduct or Performance. Within the Health directorate, a Medical Screener assesses the referral. The Medical Screener is a member of the Council and usually a psychiatrist, as most problems relate to mental health and addiction.

The Screener decides whether the information suggests your fitness to practise might be impaired and if so, the case is then dealt with under the Health Procedures. The Screener can decide not to proceed if adequate local measures are in place that both support the doctor and protect patients.

The central feature of the Health Procedures is a medical assessment by experts. Two GMC examiners assess you. You are entitled to nominate other doctors to examine and submit reports. I requested my GP and a local Professor of Psychiatry.

The initial contact from the GMC instructs the doctor to notify them within seven days of all their current employers.

The Examiners are asked by the Health Screener to provide specific recommendations on certain areas. These include whether the doctor is fit to practise, with or without supervision, on a limited basis or within certain grades or specialties. From these recommendations the doctor is invited to agree to certain restrictions. These generally ensure that the doctor does not work alone or unsupervised, in single-handed practice, as a locum, as well as restrictions on prescribing, the number of sessions worked, the use of over-the-counter medication and alcohol.

The Examiners recommend a Medical Supervisor. The Medical Supervisor may be an Examiner, or a local psychiatrist who has agreed to provide this service to the GMC.

The Health Screener reviews the reports and recommendations. The Screener asks the doctor to agree to Medical Supervision and the restrictions on his/her work. The Supervisor meets regularly with the doctor and reports to the Screener. The Supervisor also contacts the doctor's employers and whoever is supervising the doctor's medical work.

If the doctor does not agree to above conditions, fails to keep to the restrictions or their health deteriorates, s/he is referred to the Health Committee.

Health Committee

The Health Committee consists of nine members, seven medical and two lay members. All are GMC members. The doctor is entitled to legal representation. The Health Committee can ask for more evidence, suspend registration for one year or place conditions on registration for up to three years.

Each year approximately 10% of doctors under supervision are able to have their supervision concluded.[1]

You can appeal within 28 days to the Judicial Committee of the Privy Council against the decision to suspend registration or impose restrictions, but only on a point of law.

Confidentiality

Unlike the GMC's Conduct procedures, the Health procedures are conducted in private. However, by law the GMC is required to inform your employers, the Department of Health, the Scottish Office and National Assembly for Wales of the procedures and restrictions, as well as anyone inquiring about your registration. The Medical Supervisor discusses your health and work performance with your work supervisor, your GP and your psychiatrist.

Further information

The GMC will provide information about the procedures through their Fitness to Practice Directorate. The GMC produces also produces a booklet *Helping Doctors Who Are Ill*.

The GMC advises contacting your defence organisation as soon as you are informed you are being investigated. They were a valuable source of advice to me.

Support organisations, e.g. the Doctors' Support Network, can put you in touch with other doctors who have had similar experiences.

The BMA offers general advice and support.

How to survive

The GMC process erodes self-confidence and self-belief. It is very threatening and isolating. The underlying mental health problem must still be managed. Staying well and fit for work are a daily battle for someone with serious ongoing illness, without the added struggle of the GMC Health Procedures.

A crucial factor in my survival has been a very supportive and proactive GP and a new psychiatrist. The above process had very damaging effects on the relationships with both my GP and previous psychiatrist. Although my GP was involved in the initial referral and still feels requesting advice was the right decision, the subsequent process she has found horrifying, bewildering and frustrating. It is ideal if it is your psychiatrist and GP that provide support for you and represent your needs with the GMC Screener. This leaves you able to manage your illness and continue working if appropriate.

It is worth asking whether specific restrictions can be revised or reconsidered if you, your GP and psychiatrists feel that they will adversely affect your health and employment. I requested that the letter sent to my employers stated that I was complying fully with the procedures and that I was being carefully monitored by my GP.

I was concerned about my medical confidentiality and my employers. I therefore arranged for an educational supervisor (my GP trainer) to liaise between the Health Screener, Medical Supervisor and my employers. This has worked well.

Once the supervision starts, the Medical Supervisor can be contacted if there are specific problems relating to the restrictions and your working practice.

Continuing with normal activities and a structured week helps keep the GMC investigation in perspective. I also found peer support and sharing the experiences of other doctors helpful. This came mainly from the Doctors' Support Network.

For the future

I found the above process very frightening. I felt isolated. The sense of guilt, shame and failure that was already a debilitating feature of my illness increased enormously.

It was very formal, and the special delivery of legal-style documents was very threatening. Some of the threat and subsequent anxiety would be eased if the approach were more personal. I received standard letters that were intended to protect patients from the worst scenario of addiction and ill health, rather than relating to my own case. Being a doctor is a vital and integral part of one's person; it is rarely just a job. Going through and still being under the Health Procedures hit my whole being very hard.

Doctors subject to the Health Procedures are assigned a caseworker. It would be more helpful if the caseworker could provide specific support and information to the sick doctor. He/She could introduce themself to you when the initial referral was received and explain in advance the next step, e.g. 'You will receive a standard document in the post asking you to agree to be examined by two . . .'.

Ultimately I feel it would be better if the Health Procedures were separated from the GMC. There is clearly a conflict of interests between the need to protect patients yet respect the confidentiality and rights of the doctor.

The GMC must protect patients, regulate the profession and investigate the conduct and performance of certain doctors in order to do this. The GMC's Health Procedures are too closely linked with those for Conduct and Performance. At present the health of sick doctors is investigated and regulated in a similar manner, by the same organisation.

There is a pressing need for openness and acceptance of ill health in doctors. Without this the public cannot be protected adequately. The current system relies on referral from colleagues and employers together with self-referral. It would be more effective and less prejudicial if the service were separate from the GMC and run by an independent body. The Faculty of Occupational Health is the obvious choice. Occupational Health Physicians are employed in industry, the armed forces, insurance companies and most of the NHS to monitor the health and fitness of employees. The Occupational Physician examining and advising the sick doctor could refer to the GMC should their recommendations be ignored.

Reference

1   Sheila Mann (2000) Cases considered by the health screeners. Report to General Medical Council, Annex A Table 3. April.

Summary

- The GMC procedures are designed to protect patients and help a sick doctor. Whether they do this is a point for debate.
- Managing your illness and dealing with the procedure, which undermines confidence, is demanding.
- Support from health professionals and medical protection organisation is vital.
- Peer support is helpful.
- Linking health issues with professional misconduct by having the GMC deal with both adds to the shame attached to the Health Procedures.
- Health Procedures should be completely separate from disciplinary procedures.

Chapter 21

Reflections on illness and health

Petre Jones, Joanna Watson, Helen Johnson, BS and Anon

Poetry looks at things differently from prose. We have drawn this selection from the many which were submitted to us, not because they are necessarily well written – although many are – but because they speak about what it is like to be a doctor and be troubled by mental illness. They cover a wide range of feelings, from despair to relief and joy. So dip in and let them speak to you of people's experience.

The rope

The rope hung invitingly over the neat brick wall of medical school.
A grab.
Missed.
A grab again
and the ensuing steady ascent was acknowledged
adequate
in the qualifying rounds.

Now real climbing began in earnest.
Six- or twelve- month cycles of dogged training
trusting a new rope,
tackling a different rock face,
learning to ignore the fear of the sheer of the sheer drop below
while holding onto narrow ledges of exhilaration.

The challenge of an overseas climb,
considered by some to be the Olympics of them all,
was carefully planned.
begun,
failed.

Gentle climbs back home
now loomed like Everest
each tackled,
conquered.

Then the stumbling began.
Footing missed over and again.
One day, part way up a precipice
the feet lost hold.
And no sign of the rope.   *Anon*

Doctors with attitude

Ranked high among gods
we drink the oblation of devotees
flavoured by
obedience   'sign the consent form here'
service   'a few more days yet, Mrs Smith'
and daily penance   'take two every night'
spiced with their unswerving faith
that such human sacrifice
earns relief from distress
of body and of mind.

But let us not forget,
we to whom such worship is addressed,
this cup from which we quench our thirst   so professionally
holds ingredients past, present and yet to be.

Anon

On admission to hospital

Small dense sphere of darkness
tightly packed with nothingness,
magnet for the detritus of the world
imploding on impact.

Anon

My room at hospital was not well appointed

My cell is bashed-up blue, cold and empty,
A hardboard curtain on a broken perspex window
Looks out onto cell blocks C and D.
A creaky iron bed, grey duvet
And atmospheric light neither on nor off
Create the perfect gloom,
The perfect home for a depressed heart.

Petre Jones

Visitors

Why do they want to come?
To gawp, to stare, to gloat at my defeat?
I want to hide from normal eyes.
No human eye should have to see
The dilute shafts of empty light
That leak out from this dire captivity.

And yet they want to come
To talk, to share, to hold the light for me.
I'm broken down in life's pit, stopped,
And in my broken state they see,
With X-ray vision probing deep,
The still beating heart, and my enduring humanity.

Petre Jones

weekend on call

3am
Monday chilly theatre eerie blear
I scrub myself awake with disinfectant

masked gowned gloved we play our rôles
to clinical perfection

orchestrated by the surgeon Mr B Incisive
known to cut thrust sew
as many -ectomies and -otomies and -plasties as he can
at any hour and private plumbing in particular
his eyes are probes his tongue a scalpel

as he quips anatomy I grip retract
the grind of teeth the scrape of steel
a soporific respirator
monitors
my thoughts of sleep
       * * *

on Friday seventeen admissions and a Twix
then plastic cheese in swabs of sandwich snatched on Saturday
between the rounds and bloods and bleeped demands and people in distress
their lives depend on my precision   mine   in pounding
wards and lime-green corridors

becoming Sunday rain
must sign must phone must diagno—
emergencies and charts and tests
a death a drip a new admiss—
no time to sweat or feel or bed or

10pm I pause   and
bl*** that morbid-grey contraption summons me again to casualty
a tawny woman fifty with a bloated cardigan
apologises vomits writhes in pain
I stroke her hand
       * * *

and now she snoozes on the table
sterile drapes expose her
skin   slit open
bleeding   singeing arteries
her son outside

and yellow
spilling from the woman
rotting tissues mottled liver   irreparable
      we stitch her up in layers

the smell of burning human flesh

Joanna Watson

First published in *The Rialto,* Summer 2000

Pyjama people

Tranquillised stripes
slipper between sea mist and smog,
stubbed stares, grey coughs
caught in a bell-watch web.
They paddle the daily straits,
slop out nightmares,
trawl exchanges.
Seasick in sallow waters,
they drift again . . .
moon-shadows becalmed.

Schizoid checks
dance in the billows,
bellow-pump the ocean spray,
chisel the horizon
till lightning subdues them.

Unpatterned misfits
harbour silent insolence,
dark currents of shame.
Faded, wrinkled, with fraying cords,
their leggings sink, leaving
purple tidemarks.

Joanna Watson

Reprinted with permission from Elsevier (*The Lancet* 1997, **349**: 1632)

To be a patient

Place of safety so I hope,
Anger rises, fear, how to cope,
Reassuring staff try to explain,
Knots of confusion fill my brain.
Longing for peace and a head that's clear,
Am I going to discover these things here?
Now all is a journey, we have much to face,
Determinedly onwards, no winners in this race,
So each for themselves and at their own pace.

BS

Lithium

You offer me pills
To palliate pain
But my pain is not physical
Or even emotional.

My soul cries out
To be let free,
To express itself,
Be allowed to be.

No doubt your pills
Would 'stabilise' things,
Would dampen the highs
On which I fly

And drag up the lows
In which I cry,
Return me to work
And 'enable' me.

But you make me a prisoner
Of your tiny world,
You clip the wide wings
On which I see more

Because passion
And pain are the
Person I am,
The essence, the core.

And the job is a role
I took on, long ago.
It is not who I am,
Just the person you know.

So keep your pills
And let me go free.
No longer a doctor
But created to be.

Anon

Anger

Don't tell me what I feel
Or why I feel it.
Don't speak words for their sound,
I am deaf ears.
Give me the time
To draw a little breath,
Clear me a path
To leave without a fall.
They say that time heals wounds
As deep as this one.
That I will smile at
Everything lost here.

Anon

Understanding

How could you possible know
What I've been through?

I faced death,
Unafraid,
But for the pain it would cause you.

And how could you possibly know
How hard I've fought

To carry on,
Be here,
To think it through?

Pray God you will never know.
That it will not happen to you.

Anon

Kevin's poem

When you wonder if you matter to anyone at all,
if they care enough about you to approach the stony wall
of silence you've erected, to keep the world at bay,
and yet, deep down, you really hope someone will find a way
to see through the defences to the person there inside,
the one who needs affection, the child you try to hide;
who needs to sit on someone's lap, and be held tight and hugged,
who needs the reassurance of knowing they are loved;
then come and find the child in me that's also full of fear
that nobody would miss me if I were no longer here,
and as we hold each other close, we'll both see that it's true
that somebody would miss me, and that somebody is you.

Helen Johnson

In the moonlight

We stand
face to face:
you scan
my dimpled fat;
I scrutinise
your shrivelled frame
and penetrating eyes
afraid of me staring at you
staring at me.
Sallow echoes.
You catalogue blemishes;
I dream of perfection.
Miss Taken and Miss Shapen
captured in a mirror,
tortured by shadows.
Waxing and waning
reflections.

Joanna Watson

First published in *the magazine*, 1996, **2**: 49.

New dawn

A new shoot has arisen in my heart
Long forgotten and unnamed
Choked and ripped by razor thorns or
Sodden beneath wet mossy clumps or
Squashed by leathery brassicas past their seed.

A new shoot has arisen quiet and strong
Peachy soft and pastel bright
Promise of a flower to reach
The parting clouds that stretch the neck.
The fragrance quickens memories.

Warm love and boyhood fun
Honeymoon and new births
Cambridge and Lakeland
A mad guitar on Risborough's train.
The dawning shoot named Happy.

Petre Jones

Bulimia nervosa is something of an enigma. Its powerful, clandestine rituals may cause sufferers extreme distress; and others an equal measure of perplexity. From the outside, the eating disorder appears as bizarre as a poem written in neologisms. However, those who dare to look and listen within will find that the cycles and symbols of bulimia nervosa need not be totally incomprehensible.

Sublimia neovosa

e-m-p-t-i-h-o-l-e-n-e-s-s
    plinges bleakingly
        seekingly huggiful
           solone

doof plurges
    smiggles platefully
        forkward osward gutward
           accelerogobbelo
        enterotangling
    vainful pluggles
        stormcrash stormache
           borborhythmic screaks

        guttling[+++]
BLOATFULNESS
    franic exguttling
madnauseam . . .

e-m-p-t-i-h-o-l-e-n-e-s-s
    solone

Joanna Watson

First published in *Psychopoetica Introducing Poetry* 1996, **35**: 36.

Part Three

Dealing With It

Chapter 22

Ongoing support and relapse prevention

Petre Jones, Belinda Brewer and Anon

Keep on keeping on

Walk on, Walk on and on,
Whilst North wind frozen marrow
Weakens heavy limbs.
No rest, nor sleep,
Lest blood and breath dry up
Humanity like desert dust dispersed.

Yet by this evening
Warmer rays return.
False dusk-time dawn, for
Morning brings the cold wind's desert back.
And so we trudge,
Diurnal lurching, trailing pain.

The ones I love are scarred,
And yet they love,
And follow my destructive path.

With time's time passed the wind is eased
Trees and birds and air fill up
The cold dark vacuums in my mind.
The dawn is here, the world is fresh,
Freedom, colour, strength, new purpose,
But still new dawns lead round to night,
The storm waits only to return when
Happiness should fill my loved one's eyes.

This bastard illness bides its time,
Bruised by treatment, licking wounds.
We will do battle on another field,
So I lay bunkers, train and watch.
I'm waiting for it this time and will work
Till future deserts bloom and winds are warm.

As our stories show, many people's experience of mental illness is of a one-off
episode, from which they recover, to return to a changed but normal life, leaving

an ongoing sense of vulnerability. For others, with diagnoses of bipolar and recurrent affective disorder and eating disorder in particular, there is an enduring problem of recurrence and relapse. This poem expresses the morale-sapping relentless switchback of diurnal variation during an episode of illness and the enduring knowledge that at some point the illness is going to return. This chapter deals with these ongoing issues of how to keep going, enlist support and reduce the risk and damage of future episodes of illness.

Learning a new self-identity: a personal story

When I first became depressed at the age of 21, I knew who I was. I knew what I thought, what I believed, how I related to others, how I saw the world. I was intelligent, confident and had friends. Then I became depressed. Suddenly, I was no longer the capable person I had thought I was. I was no longer in control of myself – simple actions like getting out of bed suddenly became equivalent to doing a marathon. I did not recognise this being which hid under the duvet, desperately clinging to a teddy bear, crying for hours at a time. I couldn't cope with basic decisions such as what to wear. I wanted people around, yet could not cope with holding a conversation. On the days when I did function, I only did so by talking myself through each step of the way, as if programming a robot. And through it all was the isolation – sometimes a fog, usually a glass case surrounding me, and at the bad times, a black hole with seemingly limitless depths.

As the depression took hold, it became impossible to see anything good in myself. Surely I was the worst person on the face of the planet. How could anyone tolerate me? I couldn't tolerate myself. In fact, the world would be better off without me, and I would be doing everyone a favour if I killed myself.

Gradually, things improved, with medication and a lot of support from friends. But it left me wondering who I was. What was left of 'me'? A lot of underlying assumptions about who I was had been shaken. I felt as if I was in the aftermath of an earthquake – so much devastation, but some buildings still standing (But are they safe? Can they be left, or do they need to be demolished?) – but where do you start? Not knowing who you are is a very vulnerable place to be.

I still saw the depression as something external, something which had damaged me, but would go away again, leaving me to pick up the pieces and rebuild my life. In the 10 years since then, I have had two further episodes, and probably need to stay on antidepressants for life. Having lived with depression for so long, I am no longer sure what is 'me' and what is 'depression'. I can usually identify a new flare-up, as I recognise my warning signs. But in between, when I am 'OK', the depression is still there in the background, even though I am not actively depressed.

Perhaps the most obvious sign of this is my 'negative filter'. When I am actively depressed, this comes out in full force. It is as if everything passes through this mental filter before reaching me. So if someone says 'You're looking good today', what actually comes through my negative filter is 'You looked awful the last time I saw you'. When I am 'OK', the filter is still there, but much less obviously. This can make it difficult for me to know if I am over-reacting to a situation because my negative filter has interpreted it wrongly, or if the situation genuinely demands a certain reaction. I know there are certain topics which I do better to avoid, because they bring my filter out in force, and so I tend to be much more careful of my reaction if one of these topics is involved. Feeling that you cannot rely on yourself to interpret the world accurately is quite difficult to live with. I cope with it by 'reality checking' – asking someone else what they think about it. At times I forget the filter is there, but then I say something which brings other people up short, and I realise that I see the world from a slightly skewed viewpoint, which seems to be different to how most other people perceive it.

Oddly enough, I am now much more extroverted than before I got depressed. I am still temperamentally an introvert, and need quite a lot of time and space to myself, but I am much more outgoing than before. I have also learned that I need to look after myself, and that saying 'no' to other people is not a crime. I am still working out who I am, and I know that I will always seem slightly odd to some people. I think the biggest change has been the loss of certainty – I always thought it would never happen to me, and it did.

Anon

Knowing oneself and the illness

The prime responsibility for dealing with the illness lies with the patient, and for many of us it has been helpful to draw up a relapse prevention plan. This is based on knowing our own illness, how we tend to present at different stages of severity and what behaviours we tend to display and symptoms we experience at each stage.

The precise early warning signs will vary between people, and so in this chapter we have tried to include severe different people's experience.

My personal signs

Early warning signs that I try to recognise in myself vary depending on whether my mood is dropping or elevating. It has taken about six years for my GP, friends and I to identify these. As I become depressed I begin to withdraw from colleagues, friends and neighbours, answering the phone or dealing with the mail becomes increasingly difficult. I am generally angry and irritable and this is disproportionate to the situation. Involuntary, intrusive suicidal thoughts distract me; my GP has noticed I wear more perfume.

As I become more hypomanic I become louder and I tease people. I spend more money on non-essentials and everything seems to sparkle. I am particularly drawn to silver items. Eighteen months ago I located a silver

Audi A3 on the Internet, about 100 miles from my home. I arranged to meet the dealer at a service station on the M3 where I bought it on a Visa card.

It is much easier to recognise the early signs of depression, it is horrible and you want the feelings to go away. You are more prepared to make changes to work, lifestyle and medication. Unfortunately the early signs of hypomania often feel great. You are a fun person to be with, have loads of energy, are very motivated and productive. Understandably, making changes at this stage is much harder and less likely to be seen to be necessary.

Belinda Brewer

Having identified patterns that suggest illness, one can add in actions to take if one recognises the illness returning. An action plan can be shared with family and friends and professionals to give them clues on how to help.

An example of an action plan for someone with recurrent depression

Recognising the illness
The symptoms at each stage of the illness are based on what it has been like for this person in the past, and particularly those symptoms that they can recognise.

Normal
- One tired day does not make depression.
- Accept normal anxiety and mood variation.

Mild illness
- Tired most of the time.
- Not talking so much with family in evening.
- More than usual bad moods with the kids.

Moderate illness
- Bad tempered and irritable at work.
- Persistently tired.
- Poor sleep at night.
- Suicidal thoughts not intrusive or dwelt on.
- Self-harming for release.

Severe illness
- Diurnal variation.
- Early morning waking.
- Stiff face and limbs.
- Struggling to keep up at work.
- Intrusive suicidal thoughts.
- Self-harming for self-hatred.

Very severe
- Suicidal planning and gathering tools together.
- Psychotic-like experiences, e.g. bizarre experiences, paranoid thoughts.
- Escalating self-harm for hatred.

Action plan

Actions are based on what is possible for the patient at each stage of the illness.

Normal

Maintain regular medication and contact with CPN and psychiatrist.

Mild

- Time to dust off CBT skill again.
- Prioritise work, no new projects.
- Discuss with CPN and psychiatrist at next visit.

Moderate

- Tell spouse and key support people including CPN.
- Reduce work and home load.
- Post on DSN site.

Severe

- Consider time off work.
- Bring forward psychiatrist or GP appointment.
- Avoid being alone in surgery.
- Intensive CBT skills.

Very severe

- Contact or ask someone to contact psychiatrist today.
- Alternatively, see GP today.

The whole point of the relapse prevention plan is to help the patient and others take action early and appropriately, before ideas of lack of self-worth or inappropriate hopefulness tell the patient that it's not worth getting help now. 'You're not really ill, you're making it up.' 'Don't make a fuss about nothing.'

The plan can be as complex and obsessive as you wish, including trigger factors and danger times, and details of who in the informal support network might be appropriate to contact in different situations.

Another example of a relapse prevention plan, looking at fitness to practise

I am a GP with depression. I have been on antidepressants for the best part of 10 years. I know when the depression is getting worse, as I start finding it harder to get through the day, and feel emotionally more fragile. However, I usually push myself to continue working, even when I know it is not in my best interests to keep working. I hate going off sick with anything, as it means increasing the workload on colleagues, but I particularly hate going off sick with depression. Regardless of what I try to tell myself, I feel there is a stigma associated with having depression, but if I have had minimal time off work then it lessens the stigma.

My warning signs that I need to organise some time off

- Feeling it is more difficult to make decisions.

- Worrying about decisions (particularly if I do this at home, after I've finished work).
- Double-checking everything.
- Feeling my brain is slowing down.
- Panicking at the thought of doing a surgery.
- Having to consciously talk to myself before each patient comes in, to tell myself 'it's all right, you *can* cope'.
- Eating chocolate at every opportunity.
- Yelling at reception staff when they ask me to do something when I am trying to do something else.
- Finding it difficult to prioritise or deal with more than one thing.
- Throwing the bleep across the room and swearing at it when it goes off during the evening (I think this is normal behaviour at 2am).

My warning signs that I need to be off NOW!
- Bursting into tears between patients.
- Crying in the car between home visits.
- Feeling that I cannot think in a straight line.
- Finding decisions almost impossible to make.
- Thinking about self-harm and finding where the scalpels are kept.

These signs are peculiar to me, and it has taken a while to recognise them.

Anon

Who is appropriate to help pick up early warning signs?

Professionals: GP, psychiatrist and mental health team (if involved in your care). The likelihood of early signs being picked up by professionals depends to a great extent on how often there is contact. In the early stages of a relapsing illness it may be best to negotiate regular contact and easy access to a professional.

The role of relatives, friends and colleagues is very difficult. Personally I (BB) have found it extremely difficult to involve my family. It is natural to want to shield those close to you from the pain of seeing you ill. I think it is similar for friends, with the added worry that they will not want to continue the friendship once they have seen you ill. This has only happened to me on two occasions.

Colleagues are different. Trusting a colleague with details of your mental health and signs of deterioration is extremely hard and possibly not a good idea. My experience (BB) is extensive, I have worked in medicine, palliative care, A&E and General Practice. I have always been open and frank about my illness when applying for jobs. At this stage most employers have still been keen to employ me. Unfortunately when I have become unwell and need time off at short notice or significant modifications to my timetable there has not been enough slack in the system. I am very different when depressed, angry, irritable and anxious. Colleagues and senior doctors have understandably found this too difficult. If you are explicit to colleagues about the signs that you are becoming unwell, this leaves you very vulnerable. There is obviously the fear that colleagues will report you as unfit and this will have a negative effect on your future career.

I have listed all the negatives about being open to colleagues. If you can find an employer and colleagues that can put into practice all the assurances made when you are well, this is ideal. It is rare. I currently work in a GP practice that is very supportive. I have not been explicit about my early warning signs. However, all the staff including fellow GPs, practice managers, secretaries, nurses and reception staff have determined these for themselves. They know probably before I do that I am becoming unwell. My workload is reduced, I am given more time for paperwork and they accept that I may need time off at short notice. PJ's experience is similar.

It is extremely important that colleagues do not get involved in the management of your illness.

Both PJ and BB find it very useful to have a plan that documents the symptoms and signs at various stages of their illnesses. It is useful for others to know what to do at these stages. It also helps them to have more insight when we are reluctant to see that we are unwell.

The last thing to say in this section is that the poem expressed something of the ongoing grind of illness.

- The up and down nature of diurnal variation, in which one goes to bed feeling better and more positive, hoping that a corner has been turned, only to wake up early next morning feeling stiff and dreadful again.
- The constant nag in the back of the mind that a recurrence is not far away, especially when one can time the recurrence pattern to a relapse every 3–4 years or so.
- The tired and wearisome recognition of old symptoms that point to a return of illness, and lead to that heart-sinking moment when one mutters 'Oh shit!'

How one gets through these moments is different for us all. For some it is the support of family and friends that keeps them going. For others there is also support and meaning in spiritual encounters and the experience of faith.

For all of us the Doctors' Support Network provides a discussion space where doctors with mental health problems can share their experience and feelings and be sure of an understanding empathic response that will tell it like it is.

Depending on others

Part of the title deeds of being human is the need to be supported by others, and for those of us with mental illness the need is not different, just writ large. It is hard to be vulnerable, especially when our professional role encourages us to take a lead and to help others rather than being helped, but be helped we must.

Formal support mechanisms are important. Elsewhere we have discussed the need to be registered with a GP. They will provide access to secondary care, regular medication, administrative functions such as certificates and insurance documents and, perhaps most importantly, provide a space in which you can be listened to and valued. Your time with the GP is your time, albeit all too short. It goes without saying that the GP should not be a partner in your practice, as this creates too many conflicts of interest, although in isolated rural areas this may not be possible. Finding and registering with a GP you are comfortable with may not be easy, so this is a time to use your inside knowledge of the system. A good GP will help with liaising with secondary care when this is appropriate for you

Mental health services will also provide ongoing support. PJ meets up with his CPN every month or so, and with his psychiatrist every three months or so when well and every month or so when unwell. He is also able to contact her, or for people to contact her on his behalf, in crises. She can arrange admission as needed.

These are the formal networks. Your own informal network will be as individual as you are. How supportive someone might be depends on your relationship with them and how able they are to deal with your illness. For some of us our spouse is the natural key supporter but for others the spouse may find it too painful, for a variety of reasons, to engage with your illness. You will need to decide who to tell about your illness and learn which of your family and friends you can be upfront with, and who will act on your behalf. As a base line function the informal network should at least be able to say to you: 'Something's wrong, have you seen your GP/looked at your action plan?'

Last point on networks. Consider the effects of your illness on others. This is hard to do when you're ill, but reflecting on it when you are well might make people's actions more understandable. It works in two ways. First, emotions resonate with those with whom we interact. So if someone has a generalised anxiety disorder, their spouse with tendencies to obsessiveness may feel their sense of order is threatened by the seemingly endless series of potential threats envisioned by the patient, leading to more anxiety in the spouse. Anxiety feeds anxiety, and in the same way other emotions resonate in other people, reflecting their inner issues. How true it is that we all have 'issues'. The result is that some people whom you might have expected to be close to you in adversity turn out to have problems with your illness and react in unexpected ways.

The second type of interaction with others is on a behavioural level. It is true of depression, and probably true of other illnesses, that it can lead to behaviours that get people's backs up. When ill, I used to hold my hands to my head and cower when criticised or challenged, in an effort to protect myself from the emotionally and even physically painful verbal attack. This was natural enough for someone feeling vulnerable, but of course the person challenging me, seeing what to them was an excessive defensive response to their comments, would be angered more by the behaviour, making the whole scenario worse. I now have learned to abandon this unhelpful defence and instead look people in the eye, or the bridge of the nose at least, which tends to make people feel listened to, and defuse anger.

I wonder if these two mechanisms of interaction with others are what lead to inexplicable breakdowns in relationships with professionals and inappropriate labels of personality disorder. Whether or not this is true, we would all do well to understand these interactions because maintaining supportive relationships is central to staying well, or at least surviving the ups and downs of enduring illness.

Some of us will never fully be free of our mental health problems, but then the diabetic and the person with heart disease also have permanent health problems. So, rather than dwell on the possibility of relapse, the 'When?' and 'Why?' and 'How bad will it be?', consider the last part of the poem that opened this chapter.

This bastard illness bides its time,
Bruised by treatment, licking wounds.
We will do battle on another field,
So I lay bunkers, train and watch.
I'm waiting for it this time and will work
Till future deserts bloom and winds are warm.

The message is simple. Be prepared, but for your future, focus on the warm and flowering times, the good times, the love and companionship of friends and family. These are the things to live for.

Summary

- Mental illness may be a one-off episode, but for some it is recurrent or enduring.
- Relapse prevention planning can help to manage a recurrence.
- Relapse and recurrent and simple diurnal variation sap morale and undermine confidence.
- Access professionals you can trust and trust your professionals.
- Build a network of friends who can say: 'You are not right, seek help now'.
- Unhelpful behaviours and difficult transferences will have an effect on family and friends.

Chapter 23

Ideas for the dark days

Joy Pope

Doctors are human and it is a normal part of being human to be vulnerable. It is also normal to search out comfort and relief when life hurts. Other chapters of the book deal with professional help. But emotional pain takes time to resolve, whether with pharmacological or talking therapies, not to mention the length of waiting lists to access such help. This chapter is about simple things which can help during these waiting times. The suggestions are intended to be in addition to, and never instead of, expert advice. I have gleaned them from my own experience of depression, from patients and from family and friends, including those in the Doctors' Support Network, who have also been in difficult places. They are relevant to dark or anxious times, whatever the cause. Most are not specific to doctors and it is unlikely that you will find every idea to be useful. My criterion for inclusion, however, has been to know that someone, somewhere has found each to be helpful.

Be honest with yourself

Many people struggling with mental illness battle with a feeling of fraudulence and disbelief in the possibility of recovery, often both at once. The fear of fabrication or of exaggerating symptoms seems to be particularly common among medical staff and can be a barrier to seeking help. It can be hard to be absolutely truthful with yourself about how you feel and what that does or does not imply.

First, it is OK to admit you are feeling rough. It is neither being fraudulent, nor being a wimp, even if you can think of someone you perceive to be worse off than you are. It is simply a fact and you cannot move on unless you admit it.

At the same time it is important to remember that the fact you feel bad now is just that, a fact about how you are feeling now, full stop. It is not a judgement or a prophecy. The fact that you may feel worthless as a person does not mean that you are worthless (judgement). The fact that you feel awful now, on this date and at this time, does not mean that you will feel like this either for the rest of today or forever (prophecy). Feeling lousy at this moment in time is enough to cope with. Take it a day or even an hour at a time.

Keep things simple

Depression often means that the things which you normally turn to for relaxation or pleasure leave you cold, and poor motivation and concentration may make them hard to do. Sometimes the result is that you feel even worse as you become acutely aware of what you have lost, or you feel unworthy of being able to enjoy anything, especially if you are off work. **This is a common experience.**

If you are feeling like this then it is best to keep things simple. Forget *The Times* crossword, the hike up the local hills or heavy medical journals. The time for them will return. Try a simple puzzle book or jigsaw, skim through a light magazine or a well-loved children's book, potter around a garden centre. Allow yourself to watch 'trash' on television, put your usually green fingers to caring for just one planter, or a single winter bulb. Use your creative talents but at a much simpler level than usual.

Keeping things simple can also make other areas of life easier, such as meals, shopping etc. If decision making is difficult then consider shopping at a small supermarket where you can get all the items you need in one go, but where there isn't too much choice. Ready prepared vegetables are expensive but may help to maintain a balanced diet. If you have children, consider taking them to places where they will be entertained, allowing you a little space. Or team up with a friend for outings. At Christmas consider buying tokens or go for all the same thing from one shop.

Goal setting can be helpful to self-esteem, but only if related to how you are feeling. If you are very demotivated you may need an extremely simple target, such as washing your face each day, so that you know you can achieve something. If you are tense or stressed you may need to give yourself permission to stay in bed for an extra hour. Keep things realistically achievable.

Keep things contained

Life often seems to be out of control when you are not well. Finding a healthy way to contain your immediate surroundings can give a feeling of control returning.

Can you try to find a place in the house that is *your* space? It may just be a chair in one corner of the bedroom. Make that small area as tidy or untidy as you are comfortable with, perhaps with a plant, candle and soft toy. A fleecy blanket or throw can also be comforting to wrap around you. Even if you live on your own, a place like this can become one where you feel safe to retreat to on bad days, or where you go to write difficult letters, or ponder life issues that seem scary.

Sorting out the house after a long period of untidiness can be daunting. Can you put all unnecessary clutter from one room into a box? When you can manage it, try putting just one item away. There is an African Proverb which says, 'The way to eat an elephant is one mouthful at a time'. Eventually the box or bag will be emptied.

Remembering all the things that need doing is also hard. You may find writing things in the back of a small notebook to be helpful. Then write down in the front those things which really must be done this week. The list becomes confined to one piece of paper rather than being a huge mountain of unknown proportions. If any one item seems impossible then break the job down into its component parts. For example, paying a bill involves first finding the cheque book, then writing out the cheque, finding an envelope, addressing it, and finding or buying a stamp before posting. Each one of those tasks may be manageable when the thought of the whole is overwhelming, so the list should reflect that. Crossing completed tasks off gives a great sense of satisfaction. Some people find the idea of a list intimidating in itself and are better finding other ways of getting things done.

Use of the senses

Our minds and spirits need nurturing. Using the senses is a potent method, but it often has to be done more deliberately when ill.

Sight – light a candle, gaze at a photo, flowers, or other items of simple beauty. Take a moment to look at the world around, use time in traffic jams to look at gardens, architecture or distant hills. Go the pretty way home from work.

Hearing – music is very potent. Melancholic music somehow makes me feel understood and comforted, until I am ready to move onto something a little more cheerful, although the frankly joyful may seem to mock my despair. Loud, crashing music is good when angry. Humming or singing softly to a favourite song can also be helpful. This is an area where everyone is very different, but can be very healing. If you have difficulty selecting which tape or disc to play then turn to your favourite music radio station to choose for you.

Touch – a warm bath with relaxing oils, soft slippers, or a fleecy rug can all be comforting. Some people find a massage beneficial, and hugs essential, while others find these uncomfortable or embarrassing. Body lotion may feel nice, or a simple foot massage. And soft toys are wonderful.

Smell – the use of lavender or other oils in a burner, a scented candle or on the pillow is a regular favourite, as is pot pourri or bath/shower oils. In work a scented hand wash can help, if you have the luxury of a room of your own. I have some good quality air freshener sprays in a couple of different scents in my surgery. I use them not only to mask odours, but also after patients with complex problems have been in, to help change the atmosphere.

Taste – most people under stress eat either more or less than normal and often not as healthily as usual. Food may not taste good or you may crave food to fill the sense of emptiness inside. Making yourself savour what you are eating may help.

Humour – comedy programmes and books of cartoons are excellent, and laughing is good therapy if you are able to. Being able to laugh when low or anxious is not a sign of fraudulence, but may be a small light in an otherwise dark sky.

Use of symbolism and the imagination

The use of symbolism and imagery can be very powerful tools. Here are some ideas, but the list could be endless.

Remember you are supported. This is particularly helpful if you are feeling agitated or having a panic attack. Become aware of all the things that are supporting your body such as the chair you are sitting on, the floor, the earth; they are holding you, keeping you. Then move on to think of people who hold you – professionals, family and friends, pets you dare to believe still care for you at such times. Allow yourself to feel supported, maybe imagining them as a safety net beneath you.

Use images or symbols of things and people that support – photos in your surgery, wallet or purse. You could try something small in your pocket to finger at difficult times, perhaps something small but given to you by someone significant to you, or conveying a memory of a special time in your life.

Devise a Yellow Bag. This was an idea I had once on returning to work from a period off ill, when I was rather unsure of myself. I decided that I needed something more than my doctor's black bag. I designed in my mind's eye a large bag in my favourite colour (yellow!). And imagined it full of reminders – a photo of my god-daughter, a bunch of flowers which someone had given me while I was off work, a friend's dog which always bounces up to me cheerfully, hugs of family and friends and so on. In between each patient I mentally opened the bag and chose one thing to remind me of the love and care which was there for me. It helped restore my smile as I imagined Charlie the dog bounding up the surgery corridor.

Keep a Pollyanna Book. This is named after the classic children's book *Pollyanna*, about a young girl who had an amazing way of finding brightness in the darkest of situations. This idea is different from keeping a journal of emotions or a mood diary. A notebook or diary with a cheerful cover is ideal. The aim is to write something positive each day, no matter how small. It may record the first snowdrop or cuckoo, a funny thing a child said, something which amused or amazed you on TV. Keep the entries short, limited to one sentence and about just one event (i.e. be achievable). It helps to remind you that life contains good as well as bad, and also can be helpful later, to remember that even in the blackness there were tiny rays of hope, even when you could not feel them to be there.

Use any symbols from your personal faith system, if any, provided they are helpful. Think about the symbolism of a candle in the darkness, a pebble smoothed by the sea, a seed growing out of the earth etc.

Mantras and similar phrases. These are particularly helpful if you are having a panic attack or having intrusive thoughts of self-harm. A simple phrase to repeat which reminds you of a helpful truth and which keeps you in the present can help. These are common in some religious circles, but they do not have to be faith-related. 'I am sitting on a chair' is a very simple example.

Relaxation exercises. These methods of tensing and deliberately relaxing each muscle group, while concentrating on slow breathing, are widely used and are often accompanied by music and imagination of the place the person feels most relaxed, e.g. a favourite holiday destination. They can induce a sense of deep relaxation and wellbeing, but may be difficult for some people, especially if very tense or agitated. Limiting the muscles groups may help initially, e.g. just relax the arms, or omit the whole of the first part and sit or lie down to relaxing music, while thinking of your favourite place.

For folk in clinical work, keep an emotional distance between yourself and your patients. This does not mean losing empathy or understanding, but finding ways to help you not to carry the burden of somebody else. Taking on yourself the hurts of another does not lessen their pain, but may make you less able to help them, as well as make it harder for you to deal with your own baggage. There are various symbolic ways of helping. Some of these will be easier to apply to the GP setting than hospital clinics, as GPs are more likely to have their own room.

- Fresh air spray. A good quality one to spray after a difficult consultation can help lighten the room and yourself in the process. Citrus scents are good for this.

- A favourite soap can do likewise. See also above about use of the senses.
- A dish of small pebbles (but not so small that any visiting children may choke on them!). Pick up one after a charged consultation and imagine the pebble having heard the story and containing it within itself. Wash it, or put it down somewhere deliberately as you, too, put the memory of that patient down. Incidentally, the pebbles can also be helpful for tense patients to finger while trying to talk about personal or embarrassing issues.
- Can you imagine a line drawn down the middle of surgery/clinic between yourself and the patient? Remember, the line is still there, even if you have physical contact with the patient, a reminder as to whom the issues belong.
- Use the room itself. Open the door or window between patients as a reminder that the patients have left, carrying their own burden, your part being to help them shed their load for themselves, to empower them where possible, not to take it off them onto yourself.
- Keep a scribble pad to hand, and scribble how you feel, using doodles or just a couple of words. Put as much emotion as you need into the writing; you cannot hurt pen and paper.
- If you still feel the weight of a patient, then acknowledge your feelings but try to break the sense of heaviness. Leave the room or ward, even if just for a moment, make contact with a nurse or receptionist, make a drink, go to the toilet, take a few breaths and remember your own supports (see the first suggestion in this section). If there is a common theme to the sort of patients which you find touching your emotions (e.g. certain forms of loss), then this is something to discuss with a counsellor or other therapist.
- A shower on going home can be used as a form of ritual to wash away lingering heaviness of the day. If you live on your own then it may be important for you to make yourself do something non-medical that evening.

Thoughts on being 'selfish' and other difficult issues

Selfish or self-love?

Most people are taught from childhood that it is a bad thing to be selfish, and many come to think of loving themselves as being in the same vein. However, I would argue that the two are very different. Most parents love their children, yet do not wish them to be selfish, but be able to look after themselves and grow as people, and also to be compassionate to others. It is no different when it comes to loving yourself. To love yourself may mean making yourself get out of bed to go to work to earn money to keep yourself and family. Or it may be to do a new course to expand yourself. At other times it means spending time with partner, family or friends to nurture their and your relationships, or having an early night to restore your batteries, or taking time off to recover adequately from a physical or emotional illness. Loving yourself means working towards the best for yourself according to the situation you find yourself in. It is vital to recovery.

Doormat or red carpet?

There is a difference in being a doormat and a red carpet. A doormat gets ignored, badly treated, and soon fills up with everyone else's dirt. A red carpet is well cared for and used on appropriate occasions only. This makes the person walking on it feel special. So with yourself. You may need to give yourself to be walked over at major crisis times, and this helps the person concerned, and enables them to go on with their lives. But if this becomes a way of life then you have become a doormat. This results in your being worn out, and those walking on you are not helped to empower themselves.

Superhuman or superwimp?

Doctors are as human as their patients. If good clinical care for a patient means professional care, why should this be denied doctors? If you are not well then it is right to seek professional help. Make that appointment with your GP – or maybe first of all register with another doctor outside your practice! You may have the knowledge base to treat someone with your condition but you do not have the objectivity. Good care generally involves the patient in decision making, but always requires an objective clinician. You deserve as good care as anyone else – it is not being wimpish.

Never say 'never'

When I was a medical student I was advised that any multiple choice question in a clinical exam that used the words 'never' or 'always' was virtually always false. Remind yourself of this if you find yourself saying 'I always get it wrong' or 'I shall never get out of this black hole'.

When thoughts of suicide and self-harm threaten

If suicidal

Thoughts of suicide come in different ways to different people. If you have had any such thoughts, no matter how vague, then it is important to have a strategy in place should they try to become overwhelming. Depression is treatable, you will not stay this way forever, despite what your thoughts tell you, and you deserve and need to be kept safe during these very dark times.

First of all, can you make yourself tell at least two people? One needs to be a professional such as a GP, Community Psychiatric Nurse (CPN) or psychiatrist, and the other needs to be someone at home or whom you know well.

Practical points

- Don't be afraid to call them more than once if they do not seem to understand how desperate you are feeling first time.
- It can be very difficult to say how it is out loud, and it can be helpful to write it

down for people. You could take the note with you to your appointment and either read it aloud or give it to your doctor to read for him/herself.

- If you have had to leave a message for someone, then remember that it is not uncommon for the best of professionals to fail to return phone calls, despite promises by receptionists, secretaries and the like. This does not mean that they have decided you are malingering or otherwise not at risk, but simply means you need to phone again. The person you phoned may not have received the message or it may have got lost and thus overlooked.

A written plan for these extremely dark times is very useful. It provides a concrete list of things to do at a time when decision making is difficult. It may be easier to formulate with the help of someone else.

Practical points

- Some people start by writing down all the simple things which they know bring them comfort (such as ideas already discussed in this chapter). This idea would serve as a reminder in case any agitation makes you forget.
- The main part of the plan, however, is a list of people to contact at whatever time of day or night you need them. Write them down, and their phone numbers, even those you know by heart. Memory can play tricks when there is a lot of distress.
- You may wish to begin with family and friends. If possible, choose a few different folk, so that if some are not in or are unable to help for any reason, you have others to try.
- Voluntary groups can be lifesavers. The Doctors' Support Line (0870 765 0001) is run by doctors, for doctors, and is useful for evenings and weekends. Samaritans (08457 90 90 90) are there for doctors as much as anyone else and should be included. They are also setting up email sites which may appeal to you.
- Professional help is always available. If you have a CPN you should add the team's number, and that of any out-of-hours provision they have set up. Your GP always has a contact number for emergencies.
- Finally, the bottom line could be going to Accident and Emergency. Decide in advance whether you would want to use your local Casualty department or head for another. You may need to choose a taxi firm to get you there, in which case look up the phone number and write this in the plan also. It may be worth keeping the likely cost of the taxi fare in an envelope with the plan.

Much of this is common sense when thought about in the cold light of a normal day. However, it is very helpful to have the list all written out in a place which is easily accessible to you day or night. Hopefully you will not need to use this information, but knowing it is there helps to reduce the fear of reaching the point where you may require it. And reducing fear may also help to reduce your chance of needing it.

Assuming all this is done, and you have sought help, take each hour as it comes. Try some of the ideas already mentioned, especially in the sections about use of the senses or symbolism and imagery. Distract yourself with simple things. Some people find it helpful to make promises that they will not do something to themselves 'today'. And then again the next day, and so on. Remind yourself again of those who love you and of the hurt you would cause by carrying out any plans. This is true, and the pain of such loss goes on.

If you are having ideas of particular methods of suicide then you could try to turn your mental picture of that method into something different, and harmless, in your mind. For example, a knife might become a paint brush, tablets turn into stones along a path, or a rope become a chocolate Curly Wurly.

Meanwhile put the means one step distant from you, enlisting the help of others where possible. Ask someone else to keep your medication, or to look after car keys. Put the hose pipe somewhere which is difficult to access. Each extra step between you and a method of self-destruction will make it harder to carry out. Going to bed can be the safest option. Do keep safe. And don't be afraid to use the list of people to phone. That is why you made it.

Other forms of self-harm

Some of the basic principles above are also helpful if you are cutting yourself or have an eating disorder. Admitting it to professionals or even family can be hard to do, but you are not alone, as these conditions are not uncommon among doctors. It may help to read about the experiences of others in Chapter 9.

Getting professional help is important, as is devising a plan for when feelings of self-harm become overwhelming. Having someone to phone is important.

If you are cutting then try to put sharp items one step away from you, for example by avoiding keeping scalpels and stitch cutters in your surgery room. Try to minimise damage by waxing or making your skin go red rather than actually cutting yourself. Silicone creams to lessen scarring and camouflage creams are available on NHS prescription from your GP provided they are appropriately endorsed. The Red Cross operates a good camouflage service.

Other symptoms

Ideas for individual disorders are beyond the remit of this book, but there are many self-help groups where you can get support. They are listed in Chapter 28.

Not all the ideas in this chapter will work for you, but they have each worked for someone, so consider giving some of them a try. And do keep safe.

Summary

- Be honest with yourself.
- Set yourself simple and attainable goals.
- Nurture your sense of self through your senses.
- Symbolism and imagery can be very powerful tools.
- Identify and challenge unhelpful thoughts.
- Plan for coping with suicidal ideas and get help.

Chapter 24

Flexible ways of being a GP

Petre Jones

I have been a full-time GP now for 14 years, and throughout that time it has always been a 'challenging time of change and opportunity' in primary care. In other words, nothing has stayed fixed and secure, and new ways of working have been thrust upon us relentlessly. One of the positive sides of this restless uncertainty is the number of opportunities for GPs to work in different ways, which might suit them better. A good example of this is the rise of the co-op and the subsequent contraction of out-of-hours care. In this chapter I want to look at some of the different ways of doing GP, and see how they may benefit doctors who are or have been ill, and also help those at risk of illness.

Income protection and critical illness cover: adequate insurance

Remember your insurance in the days of your youth!

Before we start to look at the issues in detail I want to highlight a key issue for anyone. Get insurance. Get income protection insurance or critical illness cover as a minimum while you are fit and don't think you need it, because by the time you realise you did need it no one will want to insure you and you will be stuck. This is perhaps the one piece of information I would pass on to colleagues.

Partnerships

Partnerships are the bed rock of general practice. Doctors who are self-employed, retaining a lot of control over their own destiny even under PMS and the new GMS contract, ought to be able to achieve a lot of flexibility in their working arrangements to suit their personal needs, and indeed some have. However, other partnerships can be set in stone with no flexibility in workload or work pattern, regardless of the circumstances of the people concerned. Why?

What makes the difference?

You can think of a partnership in terms of the partnership deed which forms the formal legal basis of how partners interact, or in terms of the practice policies and rotas which govern day-to-day work, but it is the partnership culture, the day-to-day experience of being the partnership built out of shared history and individual value systems, that has most influence on how flexible or innovative a partnership can be.

So, with respect to the partnership deed, my practice had a clause saying that if a partner was sectioned under the Mental Health Act they could be expelled from the practice. However, the practice who had this deed were extremely flexible, allowing an ill partner times of reduced or altered working when necessary and struck out the offending clause. The point is that the relationship between the partners is really what dictates how flexibly one can work within a partnership, not bits of paper.

One of our storytellers, BS, told how she was unable to renegotiate her workload from half time. Her partners were seemingly more willing to lose a partner than come up with a flexible solution. On the other hand, in my own situation I have been able to create a practice with extreme flexibility and support built in (see the case study of The Project Surgery story) within the context of a partnership. In my case the foundation for the new practice lay in the partnership culture.

Part-time partnerships

Under the GMS contract it is possible to work full, three-quarters, half and one-quarter time, although the times that you are available to patients have to be fixed. Under a PMS contract your availability times are a matter for the practice as long as the practice as a whole meets the specification set down in its contract. As such a PMS practice may be more flexible with working times than a GMS one, but in reality it will again be the practice culture that really dictates what will happen.

Having fixed times for sessions may be good for someone with stable needs, but this will not help if there are times when you can do more and times when you can do less. There are, however, other options which might deal even with this level of flexibility, most notably the flexible career scheme.

Buying in

This is a common anxiety with people looking to join a partnership, and if one is already ill the anxiety is magnified. However, unless the practice are very rigid, this should not be a problem. Basically, there are two issues to buying in. As a partner you will own the business, and so you will need to buy a share of the business assets and equipment.

For the clinical equipment the total value in a typical practice might be up to £10 000 per wte partner, and when a new partner joins they will buy their share from the existing partners. This is, however, a simple process that can be managed on paper by the accountants, with money going from one partner to the others over the course of, say, 2–3 years or as long as you all agree to. There is in fact no legal need for all partners to have capital shares in proportion to their profit-sharing ratios (so a full-timer in a four-partner practice will have a 25% profit share, but could have only a 10% share of the assets), and indeed a partner doesn't *have to* have a share in the assets at all.

A rather bigger problem arises with owning buildings, but again this can be dealt with. Many premises are not owned by the practice anyway, so no capital problem arises. Where partners do own the building, again there is no need for all the partners to have equal or indeed any share in the building. For stable whole-time long-term partners, owning a building and receiving money from the NHS to run it as a health service practice is seen as a good investment. Essentially the partner takes out a huge loan to buy a share of the building and then gets money from the NHS in the form of a rent, which will nicely cover the interest payments on the loan. The partner will pay off the capital part of the loan slowly, as they are able, and then when they leave they will receive back the new cost of their share, to pay off the loan that is left, and hopefully, if building prices continue to rise, there will be some cash left over. Sounds easy but if you are ill or part-time or have an uncertain future there are problems in taking out the £300–400K loan that may be needed. You may have trouble getting insurance cover for the loan if you fall ill again, and don't even think about saddling your spouse with the risk of paying off £300 000 if you fall ill and can't work so can't get the NHS rent money!

There is a way around this. Not every partner needs a building share, and many partners are happy to carry a larger share, and therefore get a bigger slice of the investment. So it should usually be possible for new partners not to invest in the building if they feel unable to. Certainly, if a partnership insisted on you buying into the building I would worry about their level of flexibility as a whole.

Salaried options and flexibility

Salaried options in general practice are relatively new, and in some parts of the UK, e.g. Northern Ireland are very rare. This is a shame, as they do hold out the promise of more flexible ways of working. I am not including the old, and now rather redundant, assistantship that was partly funded by the Red Book system. These often turned out to be exploitative and with the advent of some far better options I would not advise anyone to look at assistantships. So, what are available now?

Some examples of some of the salaried jobs in Newham:

- nine surgery sessions in a large teaching practice
- seven surgery sessions in a teaching practice with protected learning time one session per month
- five surgery sessions with protected learning time one session per month
- four surgery and three CBT sessions with protected learning time one session per month
- five surgery sessions with two educational sessions per week across two practices
- four surgery sessions and four research sessions per week
- full-time as sole GP in a primary care team for transient population e.g. asylum seekers
- variable sessions averaging three per week, working in university recess and doing a PhD in term time.

These posts are all well paid, and include no out-of-hours work. They are funded either by the PCT or by PMS practices themselves through growth money, and because the funding is delegated to PCT or practice level they can be tailored to meet the needs of the applicant as much as the needs of the service. The work does not usually include any management work so at the end of the day you just pack up and go home.

Deanery-mediated flexibility

Flexible training in hospital posts is well known, and some of our storytellers have described their experience of it, including some jealousy from colleagues. One of the less young in our group did not have this opportunity and feels her career may have been very different if she had. The scheme is run by the deaneries and provides full daytime funding for training grades to work part-time, with a minimum commitment of 50%. Contact the flexible training dean at your deanery for more details, who can negotiate with the clinical tutor. Usually Trusts jump at the chance to have an extra person on the team who is virtually free to them (they have to pay out-of-hours costs). This scheme would help someone training for general practice, through the SHO years, or specialist training through SpR years, but stops when you become a GPR. GPR posts can also be made fairly flexible, and, as all GPRs are supernumerary, most training practices will be able to work the GPR job around any needs that they have, as long as this doesn't compromise training. The GPR just needs to agree working times with the trainer, who will then inform the deanery. Pay and holidays etc. can be worked out on a simple pro-rata basis based on a 10-session full-time week. I have often changed GPR time commitments to take account of illness, three times for one GPR. Illness is also a valid reason for a six-month extension.

Once trained, the deanery can still offer some flexible and part-time options. The flexible career scheme is designed to fund people to work up to an average of 50% time but the sessions do not have to be fixed each week, as long as they on average add up to the contracted total. Thus someone with children might work more in term time and less in holiday time, or someone with a recurrent illness might work more when well and then cut down when ill.

The retainer scheme was originally set up to help women with childcare commitments to work part-time in general practice and retain their skills. A retainer can work up to four sessions in general practice, in a practice that has been approved by the deanery, and they will have part funding for their work.

The returner scheme is another way of helping GPs with different career paths. It provides refresher training funded by the deanery to people who for example may be returning to work after a few years' break due to illness.

Who to talk to

So, lots of options. I would suggest to anyone looking to make a career in general practice more flexible, to fit the demands of illness, look around and talk to people and find out what is out there.

Good people to talk to include, if you are training, trainer, course organiser and associate dean. They should between them be able to help you. I have certainly helped people come up with quite innovative solutions to their needs.

For those already trained and not working, talk to the deanery, the director of primary care at the PCT and primary care tutors.

For those in a post but unhappy, I guess talk to everyone. The fundamental decision is: do you stay and make the most of it, or leave and look for something better?

Finally, as in the case of The Project Surgery, things sometimes just happen that are unexpected and amazing. Don't close your eyes to such possibilities – read on.

The Project Surgery story

I have hinted at The Project Surgery story already. Farzana and I knew each other pretty well before The Project started both at work and in educational settings. We have similar views about medicine and life in general, and are both basically interested in people, although we are happy to disagree and remain friends. All this went a long way to creating a partnership culture that valued the individual, put colleague welfare high up against patient welfare, and was prepared to be innovative.

It came about that we were looking to leave the practice we were in at the same time. I had been recovering from an episode of severe depression that had lasted nine months and expected another full episode in a couple of years, and Farzana was expecting a baby and was quite ill. To add to that, we both had mortgages and family responsibilities.

In line with the advice above I spoke to anyone whose opinion I trusted and then went to the director of primary care. I wrote a business plan to take with us that summarised our thoughts so far. Fortunately, I had run a couple of VTS courses on business plan writing so had some idea how to do this. We had decided that to do medicine on a small and human scale required a small practice and if we were the only partners we could be as flexible as we liked. Training was important to me so we built that in.

So far so easy – on paper. We thought we might take over one of the vacant practices that were becoming free with retiring GPs, but with discussion with the director we found that either the list size was not right or the premises were not right or the retirement of the incumbent GP wouldn't happen for 2–3 years, which would mean us locuming or doing salaried jobs for quite a while. We were beginning to lose heart when he finally thought of New Deal for Communities.

This is the magic wand bit, that just happened at the right time and the right place. This was not predictable and felt truly miraculous. New Deal for Communities are a government-backed development agency aiming to regenerate, in our case, a small area of Plaistow. It also so happened that the health person at NDC was a friend of mine. It also so happened that they wanted to set up a new practice in Plaistow because at present there were lots of patients who had no access to GPs. We went to talk to NDC and it also so happened that the local housing association had just acquired a house that would be perfect as a small surgery, just a few hours before we met. Add to that a promise of £250K funding to set up and run for the first year while we built a list size. As I say, it was miraculous, and soon the house was converted and we turned our minds to how the surgery would work.

We knew we needed flexibility, and we knew we would need a skilled but supportive team. We recruited a practice manager, receptionists and practice nurse, looking particularly at their ability to support us and each other. Before we opened we had a training week and were all able to share our fears for the future and our vulnerabilities. Being upfront is a great way to teambuild and if people know what your key issues are they can work around them.

So, after one year, we now have 3000 patients, to whom we provide a patient-centred primary care service. We have 1.75 wte partners, 1 GPR, 1 practice nurse, a half-time CBT therapist, and sessional men's health nurse, benefits advisor, asylum seekers' advisor, CPN, an attached district nurse and health visitor and an art and a gardening project.

So much for the traditional care. What about the flexibilities for the staff? For reception staff, needs have been about fitting working hours around family commitments and being able to take time to take family to hospital etc. Other key staff needs have been about understanding inexperience and supported learning, being aware of and supporting through illness, and understanding personal fears. For Farzana it is largely about childcare. She felt uncomfortable leaving the baby with a childminder or nursery and her working hours would have made this difficult anyway. So instead we adapted the surgery staff room a bit and found a nanny who comes in when Farzana is doing surgery to look after the baby. At other times the whole team just chip in and look after him as required, and, surprisingly perhaps, this is not really disruptive, and is certainly good for team morale. Above all, the arrangement is very flexible.

And what about flexibilities to deal with my illness? My workload is carefully regulated. I have time specifically set aside to do management tasks, and for teaching, and I have 'down' time, one day every two weeks where I come into work, usually, and catch up a bit, or paint, or go for runs. I also find time for at least two runs per week and we have built a shower to deal with this. Running is a good way for me to relax, clear my head, think and recharge. All the team keep an eye out for me being stressed, and are all willing to listen if I've had a tough patient, for example. I get time out for appointments, including psychotherapy, and our men's health nurse practises her phlebotomy skills on doing my lithium levels. Finally, we built up a contingency fund of £20k to fund the costs of locums, in the event of another recurrence, so as to reduce the negative impact of the illness.

These are some of the practical flexibilities we have developed so far, and they arise from our partnership culture. They also depend on close trust and teamwork within the practice. We worked hard to build this by:

- All staff person specifications used at recruitment include an essential skill of being able to be supportive of colleagues within a team, and we took this seriously at interview.
- We had our training and teambuilding week before we opened to gel the team, using group-building skills learned in the course of Course Organising.
- The partnership buys food for lunch time, so the whole team can meet up in the staff room and share lunch, and childcare.

- We go out for practice evenings about every month.
- We run monthly staff meetings which are informal and either look at clinical governance and the way the practice works, or our practice education programme.
- There are regular formal and informal debrief and supervision sessions.

We are a PMS practice and one of our aims as set out in our application form is to aid recruitment and retention by adopting employment policies and practices which aim to support individual staff needs.

Obviously we have been very fortunate at The Project Surgery. We were given a building and a large sum of money at the right time, in the right place and were able to exploit our opportunities to the full. However, I believe there are lessons here for every practice if they want to be more flexible.

- It starts with the partners and the partnership culture. A couple of away-days or some facilitated meetings might explore the issues for the partnership, and make if clear if this is a way forward for them.
- Building teams is important. We have a team of about eight core people, the perfect size for group functioning. Perhaps a larger practice could break down into two or three 'practice' units, or job-based teams.
- Spend time and energy and money on the team – joint training, time together, food!
- Be imaginative in your solutions. Farzana is very good at coming up with unusual ideas, which I then turn into real solutions. Neither of us worries particularly about how things are usually done. The childcare arrangements started as a wacky idea which we didn't think could be done, until we looked in detail at how we would do it. This is the beauty of a partnership. One can do things how the partners want – within the law, of course.

Summary

- There are many career options in general practice at all levels, with partnerships, full-time and part-time, salaried options and the flexible career scheme, and flexible training.
- General practice can be made flexible if the practice culture is flexible.
- The Project Surgery story illustrates many innovative but possible ways of being flexible.

Chapter 25

The financial cost of illness

Declan Fox

I had to go off sick twice with depression when I was a full-time NHS GP and I finally had to take early retirement at the age of 44. Both spells of sick leave cost me a lot of money and my present NHS pension covers the mortgage with about £100 a month to spare.

Moral: Be prepared for the costs of illness.

But surely the NHS will look after you?

NHS employees, such as salaried GPs, hospital doctors and staff, receive full pay for six months followed by half pay for six months if they go off sick. Money is not therefore a big problem for most sick employees, because most of them will be back at work within six months, but the situation is entirely different for GPs. It is even worse for freelance or non-principal GPs.

Dealing with NHS GPs first, they generally receive their normal income (fees and allowances under the old Red Book system, now something quite different under the new contract from 1 April 2004) when off sick but they have to ensure uninterrupted provision of services to their patients and there has to be a reasonable prospect of them returning to work. If single-handed, they have to pay a locum. If in a partnership, it depends on the circumstances. A large practice may be able to manage for some time with employment of a part-time locum or perhaps no extra help at all while the other partners help with the shortfall. A smaller practice, say two or three partners, will usually need a full-time locum to cope.

A partnership, or individual partners, may have locum insurance to cover locum costs in case of sickness. Some partnerships earn a lot and are able to cover locum costs out of profits.

All locum costs are of course tax-deductible as a professional expense; monies received to help with locum costs, from whatever source, must be declared as income.

The out-of-hours co-op movement has helped a lot with overall costs; the cost of paying for a locum has gone down because there are less nights and weekends to cover. The cost per shift has gone up, of course, but not by the same factor as frequency of on-call has come down.

Any special payments for sick GPs?

Again, under the old system, some practices could claim a special sick leave payment to provide locum cover for a sick partner. This depended on the average number of patients per remaining partner. In my own case, I was in a two-man practice with around 3700 patients. When I went off, my partner was reckoned to be responsible for all 3700 and the practice was therefore entitled to help with locum cover. 'Help' is the operative word here; the payment came nowhere near covering the cost of the locum but it at least meant that I could afford the locum and have something left from my monthly cheque.

These days the situation is much more complicated; I got two different opinions in one day on whether or not the special sick leave payments still exist as a separate entity under the new GP contract or whether the payments are subsumed into the global sum. You might think you fully understand the ramifications of the new contract but you should check this out very carefully indeed.

The alternative to paying for a locum was to resign. This would have meant zero income as well as no job to return to following my hoped-for recovery. In addition, return to such a post is usually easier than going elsewhere to start all over.

Buy plenty of insurance

Moving on to freelance GPs, at the moment they have no entitlement to any NHS assistance when off sick. It follows therefore that those working for any significant length of time as locums need to be as well insured as they can afford. The first priority is income protection insurance but there are other needs like critical illness cover plus or minus mortgage protection.

The cost of most insurance is less if taken out when young and healthy. It is wise to build up a cash float (e.g. in a building society easy access account) to cover the first month or two or even three because a deferred period (meaning the time off sick before the income protection insurance policy starts paying out) reduces the costs a lot. One useful combination could be enough money in an ordinary savings account to meet outgoings for the first four to six weeks of illness, plus enough in a high-interest account for the next four to six weeks. High-interest accounts often have penalties for immediate withdrawal.

Everyone needs a good independent financial advisor; they can go through financial needs in detail and calculate the necessary level of insurance cover.

The NHS superannuation (pension) scheme – excellent value for money!

NHS employees and GPs are all members of the NHS superannuation scheme. This is an excellent pension scheme and has additional benefits like early payment of pension in case of permanent inability to return to the previous job. In my own case, I received an enhanced pension (another good feature of the scheme); it was enhanced because of my health problems and I received it because my medical attendants were able to testify that I was extremely unlikely to return to my previous work as a full-time NHS GP. There was also a good tax-free lump sum, although you should note that the actual monthly pension is taxed at source. Check the BMA website for more details and get as much advice as possible on this if you find yourself thinking of ill-health retirement. Better still, check it out with your financial advisor when still young and healthy because there are at least two ways of paying extra contributions to increase the final benefit.

Royal Medical Benevolent Fund and BMA charities

Both of these organisations can provide financial help to doctors and their dependants who are experiencing a financial crisis.

The NHS Injury Benefit Scheme – a well-kept secret?

The NHS Injury Benefit Scheme is a little-known benefit which I think is of special relevance to doctors suffering from mental illness, especially GPs. This is administered by the same Superannuation Branch which deals with your pension contributions and, once again, you will find a lot of detail on the BMA website.

Briefly, all NHS employees and all NHS GPs are eligible to claim, right from day one in their posts, if they have suffered work-related illness or injury and if they lose income as a result. The definitions of work-related illness or injury given in the English scheme booklets are actually quite wide, at least for some activities. As far as I know, work-related mental illness stands a good chance of being accepted as grounds for payment of this benefit, although applicants should be prepared for a long battle. The scheme's temporary injury benefit aims to top up income to around 85% of that received before going off sick for those who expect to return to work. Those who are unable to return to work because of their work-related injury or illness can apply for permanent injury benefit; this provides a guaranteed income and actual amount is related to earning ability. There is generally a lump sum payment for those who are permanently disabled and have had to leave their previous post as a result of their illness or injury.

Compared to the standard NHS pension, this scheme has two significant benefits for those with work-related permanent reduction of earning ability. First, for many people the payments are higher than the NHS pension. Second, they may be tax-free, although that depends on the exact circumstances.

This is a complicated scheme and if you think you may be eligible, get as much advice on it as humanly possible. The BMA pension advisors in London probably know more about it than anyone else but you do have to be a member to consult them.

I mentioned that the Injury Benefit Scheme is of special relevance to GPs with mental illness because in my experience their work is often the cause of their illness.

My own financial difficulties due to illness

Turning to my own experience again, my first spell of sick leave was for six months. When I returned, I worked three days a week for five months and did a little on-call. I was able to return to full-time work after that, although I generally hired a locum to help when my partner was on holiday and I tried to find locum cover for weekends on-call.

The following year I had a much more severe bout of depression which required specialist care including hospital admission. Onset was a few months before the acute suicidal breakdown which provoked admission and I might well have gone off earlier if not for worrying about the cost of it. On the other hand, I attended my GP and a psychiatrist, I took treatment, I had a fairly good spell most days and general consensus was that I was safe to continue working.

The weekly cost of a locum was less the second time around, due to the local OOH co-op which we started around nine months before my breakdown. The total cost was a lot more because I was off sick for around 18 months before I resigned and received my NHS pension on ill-health grounds. We were seriously worried for some time that we would have to sell our house and move to a much smaller one, but luck smiled on us, first in having some savings left, second in payouts from some de-mutualising companies, third in my wife being able to take on some extra work, and fourth in the form of an income protection policy which I took out way back. This started paying after 12 months' sickness and kept us solvent.

There is no doubt that money worries were a significant factor over the three years following my breakdown. My wife had to work extra nights on-call in her lab job to help make ends meet while I worried about return to work and earning my keep; worried that I would not be fit to return and worried that I would try it too soon. Good insurance cover and/or a prompt positive response from the NHS Injury Benefit Scheme people would have made a massive difference to my mental state. I believe that I would have recovered and returned to work more quickly if I had been assured of a reasonable income while off sick.

Summary

- Be prepared for the cost of illness.
- NHS employees get full pay for six months then half pay for six months.
- GPs who are self-employed need to get insurance.
- The NHS pensions scheme is excellent, don't leave it.
- The NHS Injury Benefit Scheme may apply to you.
- BMA charities and the Royal Medical Benevolent Society may help in a crisis.

Chapter 26

Mental health and employment

Giselle Martinez

Introduction

A recent inquiry[1] into the suicide of a specialist registrar Daksha Emson made the following observations:

- The realistic fear of stigma by Daksha and her treating professionals was a much greater driving force for actions, or lack of them, than previously allowed.
- The relationship between treating doctors and doctors in treatment requires significant attention.

Another issue highlighted as contributing strongly to the tragedy was inadequacies in NHS Occupational Health Services.

The following paragraphs will look at the state of NHS Occupational Health Services at present, government guidelines on the management of mental illness in NHS employees, your rights as an employee, career decisions and sources of advice related to employment matters.

Beyond the Clothier Report – the current political climate

The Clothier Report,[2] an independent inquiry into deaths on a children's ward caused by nurse Beverly Allitt, was published in 1994. Allitt apparently had a severe personality disorder and the syndrome of 'Munchausen by proxy'. The tragedy fed into public fears of people with mental health problems and the draft version of the report recommended that people with a mental illness should not be employed in the NHS! This was amended to include only people with significant personality disorders. It also recommended that future employees and those entering training should be screened by occupational health and not employed if they had been mentally ill within the previous two years. Active management of sickness absence was advocated since there was evidence that people with personality disorders had more brief sickness absences than others.

These recommendations led to draconian measures in some hospitals, nurses in particular being affected. Active management of sickness absence was seen as a threatening and punitive form of policing. People with disorders that made them in no way dangerous were refused employment or admission into nurse training or medical school. These measures did nothing to improve the stigmatisation of people with mental health problems and quite likely caused harm by discouraging people from seeking help from staff counsellors, clinical supervisors and occupational health.

Fortunately the political climate recently shows signs of changing in response to lobbying, disability and human rights legislation, and for reasons of practicality. Health professionals as a group have more mental health problems than the general population, and even in the general population mental health problems are common. The NHS would grind to a halt if it did not support and accept people who had been mentally ill. There is also a huge waste of public money for every doctor who is trained and then leaves the NHS.

Even before the Emson independent inquiry, the Department of Health published guidelines for managing mental illness in NHS employees.[3] Although this does not ignore the important issue of patient safety, it also stresses the importance of adequate help for staff.

The government has also launched a number of campaigns aimed at increasing morale and helping to maintain a rapidly dwindling skilled workforce. The Healthy Workplaces[4] and Work-Life Balance Campaigns[5] are examples, as well as legislation to help working parents and people with disabilities (see below).

Following the Daksha Emson inquiry,[1] the DOH in England has set up a working group to investigate the issues raised. The Doctors' Support Network has some input into this. One hopes it will be more than just a talking shop.

DOH guidelines on mental health and employment in the NHS[3]

The executive summary of these guidelines includes the following:

> . . . the stigmatisation of, and discrimination against, those who have experienced or who are experiencing mental health problems is unacceptable. . . . the NHS should take a lead, not only in caring for its present and future employees, but also in valuing diversity and in promoting good practice in the employment of people who have experienced or are experiencing mental health problems.
>
> . . . decisions relating to the employment of people in the NHS with mental health problems are to be based on a person's merits and suitability and not prejudice, irrespective of whether that person is afforded to protection of the Disability Discrimination Act 1995.
>
> A clear message is presented that, as the largest employer in the UK, the NHS should set an example showing that:

- this type of discrimination is taken seriously and will be eradicated;
- mental health should not be the cause of derision or ridicule, and;
- people with mental health problems have the same right to be treated fairly and with respect as everyone else.

General Principles laid down include:

- Selection should be based on the best person for the job. Appropriate procedures should therefore be implemented so that persons with disabilities are not placed at a substantial disadvantage compared to nondisabled persons in the arrangements made for determining who should be offered employment in the NHS;

- Every assessment for a post is specific to that situation;
- All NHS staff should have a pre employment health assessment;
- No applicant should be refused employment on health grounds unless expert occupational medical advice has been sought;
- No person should be refused employment, or have their employment terminated on mental health grounds without the NHS employer first having made any adjustments that it would be reasonable to make in relation to that person in accordance with any duty placed upon them by the DDA;
- The '2 year rule' (suggested by the Clothier Report) which some occupational health professionals have used when carrying out pre employment health assessments is no longer to be used in the NHS;
- All NHS staff need help to develop an awareness of their own mental health, when to seek help and from whom;
- The NHS needs to develop a culture where staff can be open about their mental health status, are treated fairly and are encouraged to seek help when it is needed;
- NHS managers should be aware that the DDA makes it unlawful to refuse employment or to terminate the employment of a disabled person for a reason relating to that person's disability without justification. The reason for that decision must be one that cannot be removed by any reasonable adjustment made by or on behalf of the employer.

Disability Discrimination Act

The Disability Discrimination Act (DDA) was passed in 1995 with recent amendments. It protects disabled people in:

- employment
- access to goods, facilities and services
- the management, buying or renting of land or property
- education.

For employers and service providers (e.g. businesses and organisations):

- it is unlawful to treat disabled people less favourably than other people for a reason related to their disability
- they have to make reasonable adjustment for disabled people, such as providing extra help or making changes to the way they work or can access services
- from 2004 they have to make reasonable adjustments to the physical features of their premises to overcome physical barriers to access.

For education providers, new duties came into effect in September 2002. These require schools, colleges, universities, and providers of adult education and youth services to ensure that they do not discriminate against disabled people.

Who is covered?

The Disability Discrimination Act makes it illegal to discriminate against people with a disability in certain specific circumstances, including 'mental impairment'. A person is described as having a disability in the DDA when: '. . . he has a physical or mental impairment which has a substantial and long-term adverse effect on his ability to carry out normal day-to-day activities'.

- The effect of the condition is substantial when it affects the time taken to carry out an activity or the way in which the activity is carried out, and the effect goes beyond the normal differences that exist between people.
- The effect is long-term when it has either lasted at least 12 months, is expected to last 12 months or for the rest of a person's life if shorter.
- Individuals who suffer from relapsing/recurring conditions are covered if the significant adverse effects are likely to recur beyond 12 months following the first occurrence. For example, this could include bipolar disorder or recurrent major depression where the person is well inbetween episodes lasting a few weeks.
- The definition of mental impairment currently recognised by the Act includes memory, or ability to learn, concentrate or understand.
- For recognition under the Act the mental illness has to be a condition that is well recognised by the medical profession, that is more than a mood or mild eccentricity.
- Mental health problems ranging from schizophrenia and manic depression to panic disorders and various depressive conditions are within the scope of the DDA providing they meet the requirements as set out within this definition.
- An individual whose symptoms are controlled by medication may also be covered.
- A person who has recovered from a recognised disability is also protected. For example, it would be unlawful to discriminate against a potential employee because of an episode of depression five years previously.
- These rights are only available in the workplace if the employee has informed the employer or potential employer about their condition. **This does not mean you have to tell an employer about your condition, but you can not expect their support or the protection provided by the Act if you do not.**

Employment rights are enforced through employment tribunals but employers may respond to reminders of them in an attempt to avoid these tribunals. The BMA and similar organisations would be able to offer help.

Exclusions

Certain conditions are to be regarded as not amounting to impairments for the purposes of the Act. These are:

- addiction to or dependency on alcohol, nicotine or any other substance (other than as a result of the substance being medically prescribed)
- seasonal allergic rhinitis (e.g. hayfever), except where it aggravates the effect of another condition

- tendency to set fires
- tendency to steal
- tendency to physical or sexual abuse of other persons
- exhibitionism
- voyeurism.

Discrimination and the Act

Discrimination occurs when someone with a disability is treated less favourably by an employer because of this disability, where the employer cannot show this is justified. For our purposes, therefore, it would not be discrimination if the employer acted with *justified* fears for patient safety or our own health.

Harassment (or bullying) is covered as a specific form of discrimination.

Employers have a responsibility to make sure that the way they recruit and select staff, and the conditions of employment that they offer to both new and existing staff who have a disability, do not discriminate.

Employers also have a responsibility to make 'reasonable adjustments' (see below) for employees with disabilities.

The burden of proof lies with the employer to prove he has not acted unlawfully.

Reasonable adjustments

The Act's Code of Practice[6] gives examples of adjustments that might be made for employees with a disability. The following might be suitable for a person who is mentally ill:

- Allocating some of the disabled person's duties to another person.
- Transferring the person to fill an existing vacancy.

For example, if an employee becomes disabled, or has a disability which worsens so she cannot work in the same place or under the same arrangements and there is no reasonable adjustment which would enable the employee to continue doing the current job, then she might have to be considered for any suitable alternative posts which are available. (Such a case might also involve reasonable retraining.)

- Altering the person's working hours.

For example, this could include allowing the disabled person to work flexible hours to enable additional breaks to overcome fatigue arising from the disability, or changing the disabled person's hours to fit with the availability of a carer.

- Assigning the person to a different place of work.
- Allowing the person to be absent during working hours for rehabilitation, assessment or treatment.

For example, if a person were to become disabled, the employer might have to allow the person more time off during work, than would be allowed to non-

disabled employees, to receive physiotherapy or psychoanalysis or undertake employment rehabilitation.

- Giving the person, or arranging for him to be given, training.
- Providing supervision.

For example, this could involve the provision of a support worker, or help from a colleague, in appropriate circumstances, for someone whose disability leads to uncertainty or lack of confidence.[7]

The DDA lists a number of factors to which an employer should have particular regard when determining whether it is reasonable to make a particular adjustment. These are:

- the extent to which taking the step would prevent the effect in question
- the extent to which it is practicable for the employer to take the step
- the financial and other costs which would be incurred by the employer in taking the step and the extent to which taking it would disrupt any of the employer's activities
- the extent of the employer's financial and other resources and
- the availability to the employer of financial and other assistance with regard to taking the step.

Insurance, services and premises

Apart from covering employees and recruitment practices, the DDA also covers service providers including insurance and the disposal of premises.

Service providers act unlawfully if they they treat a person with a disability less favourably than another member of the public. For example, 'A person with a diagnosis of manic depression applies for motor insurance. He is told that he will have to pay double the normal premium because of his condition. The insurer is relying on actuarial data relating to the risks posed by a person driving when in a manic episode. However, the applicant produces credible evidence that he has been stable on medication for some years and has an unblemished driving record. In these circumstances, the charging of a higher premium in this case is unlikely to be justified'.[7]

Flexible Careers Scheme

The FCS was developed as part of the Improving Working Lives for Doctors initiative. The scheme helps doctors maintain their careers by providing more centrally funded opportunities to work part-time and have temporary career breaks. The Flexible Careers Scheme funds doctors who are able to work up to 49% of full time and in each case the scheme is adapted to individual circumstances and provides sufficient medical/clinical practice for revalidation purposes. In England the Flexible Careers Scheme is managed centrally by NHS Professionals. To apply, to join or for more information, contact them on 0845 60 60 345.

In Wales, a similar scheme is called the Returner and Retainer Scheme and is managed by the Postgraduate Deanery for Wales.

Flexible training

This is discussed elsewhere.

Flexible working legislation

This legislation affects working parents only but does give some examples of the kind of working changes that may also benefit people with disabilities.

Parents of children aged under six or of disabled children aged under 18 have the right to apply to work flexibly providing they have the qualifying length of service. Employers have a statutory duty to consider their applications seriously. Eligible employees can request:

- a change to the hours they work
- a change to the times when they are required to work
- to work from home.

This covers working patterns such as annualised hours, compressed hours, flexitime, homeworking, jobsharing, self-rostering, shift working, staggered hours and term-time working.

The right enables mothers and fathers to request to work flexibly. It does not provide an *automatic* right to work flexibly as there will always be circumstances when the employer is unable to accommodate the employee's desired work pattern.

Human rights

Although the United Kingdom incorporated European human rights legislation into its own Human Rights Act in 1998, it is still possible to go to the European Court to appeal. Human rights legislation covers public bodies and services but not private organisations unless they are providing services to the public.

European human rights legislation specifically recognises the rights of people with a mental illness, including employment rights. It has a lot to say about involuntary treatment and there have been challenges by patients detained under the UK Mental Health Act.

Europe also places a responsibility on member states to take measures to eliminate discrimination against people suffering from mental disorder, raise public awareness of such discrimination and take steps promoting mental health and improving the treatment and quality of life of people suffering from mental disorder.

Occupational Health Services

Occupational Health Services vary tremendously around the United Kingdom but there is evidence that they are becoming increasingly organised and helpful. However, it is true that they are generally less knowledgeable about mental illness than they might be. They are also viewed with suspicion by many as being agents of the employer. There are also worries about confidentiality.

In fact, Occupational Health Services have a statutory role under Health and Safety legislation to give competent advice to an organisation about the safety and welfare of employees.

The DOH guidelines referred to above suggest that occupational health services and mental health professionals need to work together to provide well informed and impartial advice to managers regarding the mental health issues of NHS employees. It is advisable that treatment should be given elsewhere but that the employee should see the occupational health physician early on. The need to maintain a therapeutic relationship and the possibility of conflicts of interest mean that the occupational health physician is better able to make decisions about fitness for work, after consulting with the treating professional.

Their role will vary depending on the individual circumstances but may include:

- Helping the employee and the employer to understand whether particular behaviour observed in the workplace is related to mental health problems.
- Assisting the employee to access appropriate support through their GP, local mental health services or elsewhere, if more appropriate (e.g. if they work in the local mental health service and have concerns about confidentiality).
- Working with the employee and clinicians to facilitate a return to work through job modification and rehabilitation in the workplace.

There is also an important role for the occupational health service in the rare situation where a mental health professional looking after a healthcare worker has concerns about the safety of patients or of the individual themself and in this situation it might be helpful for the clinician to discuss the case with an occupational physician. This would certainly be the case where the patient's right to confidentiality might need to be breached in the public interest.

Any advice provided to the employer should be impartial and confidential. It could include advice on the DDA, recommended restrictions, time scales and suitable workplace adjustments.

The occupational health process – what you should expect

If you need treatment for a mental health problem I would advise consulting a GP initially. It is best not to rely on occupational health for treatment since there may be perceived or real conflicts of interest.

The DOH guidelines suggest that doctors are a special case for the reasons given above. They recommend that an occupational health service assessing doctors should be consultant-led or have access to a consultant occupational health physician.

You may self-refer if you wish, but more often the referral is made by a manager following concerns raised in the workplace. You should be told the nature of the concerns, and the purpose of referral. The OH physician should be given full details of these concerns and then make a detailed assessment of your state of health based on clinical assessment supplemented by sickness absence records, information given by the manager, and any other relevant information. A report from your GP or specialist may be sought.

The following points will need to be considered:

- The nature of the health problem including diagnosis.
- How does this affect you?
- Does this explain the observed behaviour?
- Is there any reason why you might pose a risk to others in the workplace?
- Inattention, loss of concentration, drug effects.
- Abnormal behaviours; loss of control, risk of violence.
- Degree of insight.
- Could this problem give rise to other problems in the workplace?
- Frequent sickness absence.
- Inability to make decisions, cope with emergencies.
- Seeking therapeutic relationships with colleagues.
- Is this condition amenable to treatment; is other/better treatment available?
- Is this work likely to harm your health?
- If the DDA applies, advice on suitable adjustments and time scales.

You might be referred to a psychiatrist or psychologist for further assessment. If this is for fitness to work purposes rather than for treatment, it will be a private referral funded by the employer and the nature of the referral should be made clear to you.

When OH prepares a report they should be able to advise managers in non-medical terms without breaching confidentiality of the exact nature of your condition.

OH has a key role in helping you recognise any problems and support you in them, for example facilitating out of area referrals where appropriate to maintain confidentiality.

The DOH recommends they should encourage managers to be flexible in helping you manage your time and needs *in a way that works best for you*.

Too many occupational health services are still poorly trained and poorly staffed but doctors can take the lead in demanding improvements along the lines suggested by the DOH itself. If a sick doctor considers he has been unfairly treated by OH he can request help from organisations like the BMA or the Disability Rights Commission.[8]

Career planning

It is clear from all the above that your employer has a responsibility to help you manage your career in such a way that you can continue to work despite your disability. Unfortunately there are few sources of advice available to doctors who believe a career change or changes in work pattern might be helpful. Commercial organisations that claim to help people assess their suitability for various careers are often too generalised, expensive and based on rather dodgy personality tests. One organisation that some people have found helpful is Medical Forum.[9] It may be possible to get a deanery referral. Some occupational health physicians are well informed and approachable, as are some postgraduate deans, Royal College advisors and clinical tutors. Sometimes problem-solving sessions or cognitive therapy with a psychologist might be helpful to identify particular sources of stress. Senior colleagues may be helpful but all too often they have unhelpful prejudices about mental illness.

My advice is to first find out as much about your condition as possible and try to identify areas of your work that are stressful or may cause a deterioration in your condition as well as areas which you find particularly enjoyable, stimulating or therapeutic. Ask friends, family and colleagues to help if you can, since they may notice patterns you don't. Enlist the help of a therapist if you wish. Make tentative approaches to some of the people mentioned above, without giving too much away at first. This will help you decide who is knowledgeable and likely to be sensitive and supportive. You want someone who can give you good but realistic advice and help you find individual solutions rather than off-the-peg answers. When you have decided, have some long talks, but remember: do not be rushed into any decisions, do not go back to work before you are ready and never make important decisions while you are depressed or otherwise unwell. Be brave, be assertive. Remember you are an important, expensive professional and the NHS needs you. You may, however, decide you don't need the NHS!

References

1   North East London Strategic Health Authority (2003) *Report of an independent inquiry into the care and treatment of Daksha Emson MBBS, MRCPsych, MSc and her daughter Freya*. North East London Strategic Health Authority, London. Available at: www.nelondon. nhs.uk/documents/de_inquiry_report.pdf.
2   Copies of the Clothier Report (The Allitt Inquiry) are available from The Stationery Office.
3   DOH (2002) *Mental Health and Employment in the NHS*. Available at: www.dh.gov.uk/ assetRoot/04/01/48/41/04014841.pdf.
4   Health and Safety Executive: www.signupweb.net.
5   Department of Trade and Industry: http://164.36.164.20/work-lifebalance.
6   Disability Discrimination Act 1995: www.drc-gb.org.
7   Taken from the Disability Discrimination Act 1995 Code of Practice on www.drc-gb.org.
8   www.drc-gb.org.
9   www.medicalforum.com.

Summary

- The Department of Health is starting to recognise the needs of employees with mental health problems.
- The Disability Discrimination Act, though new and largely untried, provides a wide framework for protection.
- Human rights legislation may be relevant to employees.
- Occupational health services vary but are there to help.
- Career planning advice is available sometimes.

Chapter 27

Doctors' Support Network

Lizzie Miller

DSN

Somewhere to come to when I need to be heard.
When all those around miss the sense of my words.
Expectations, agendas, they get in the way.
Obscuring the truth I am trying to say.
Trying to make sense of what happens to me,
Reliving my crises for all there to see.
Scrawling pages and pages of scribble and screed
While others go quiet in their times of need.

Reading from others their stresses and fear.
Hearing the pain that 'real people' don't hear.
Flashes of insight for them, and for me.
Writing replies that must end with a plea:
'If I am wrong and that causes you pain',
'If I am right, and that hurts just the same'.
Forgive me, bear with me, allow me to be
wrong; but accepted for just being me.

Knowing that others feel as I do.
Knowing that others have made their way through.
Hope for the dark times; someone is there
Reading my words, knowing they care.
Support freely given, not owed or deserved.
Unconditional love – yes love is the word.
Thank you for being there late in the night.
Thank you for helping me stick with the fight.

Anon, GP and DSN email network member

The Doctors' Support Network is a voluntary sector 'self-help' organisation set up to provide a forum for support and contacts for doctors who are or who have been suffering from any sort of mental illness. This chapter talks about some of the things DSN does, apart from write books, and some of the ways we have been on our journey. All royalties of this book will go to DSN rather than to the authors.

The Doctors' Support Network has two driving principles: for members to know they are not alone and to learn to be kinder to themselves and others. The group provides a safe place where doctors can be themselves, be honest about how they feel and the experiences so as to be able to overcome the isolation of mental ill health. It is a place where we do not need to pretend to be someone or something that we are not. The culture of medicine encourages us to be self-critical. Learning to be kinder to ourselves means stopping the inner voices that tell us how we should behave and what we should have done, and replacing them with a voice that asks, 'so, what did you do right and what did you learn?'. It means treating ourselves as though we are our own best friend and learning to encourage ourselves and celebrate our achievements.

The DSN offers monthly meetings in London, Bath in the South West, Cardiff, Chester and Scotland. There is a monthly newsletter, an email forum and a Support Line. The newsletter records the discussion in meetings, provides information on courses, includes telephone numbers to gain support and frequently includes articles about members' experiences of health and illness.

The Doctors' Support Line (DSL) is the telephone service open to all doctors practising in the UK, whether they are struggling with personal problems, work relationships or work problems. It developed from a collaboration between the Doctors' Support Network and the charity PriMHE (Primary Care Mental Health Education). It currently opens for 36 hours a week, and is run by volunteer doctors. The volunteer doctors have been trained to listen actively and interact with the doctors who call. Instead of a doctor–patient relationship the caller and volunteer relate to each other as peers and fellow medics, the volunteer offering the caller options rather than advice. The Doctors' Support Line also has an Information Resource, which contains basic information about services that are available to doctors. This includes topics such as information about the Sick Doctors' Trust for doctors with addiction problems, the Medical Benevolent Fund, which provides financial support for those doctors unable to work and receiving state benefits, as well as information about Occupational Health and the Disability Discrimination Act.

Seven years ago, the DSN began its life as an advertisement in the back of the *BMJ*. Dr Soames Michelson had come through a period of depression. During that time he felt totally isolated from all other doctors, believing that he was perhaps the only doctor who had ever been mentally ill. When he recovered from his depression, he remembered this feeling of being completely alone and the feeling of shame at having let the profession down. He realised that he could not have been the only doctor to have a mental health problem. He put an advertisement in the *BMJ* asking if there were any other doctors who had also had mental health problems. I and over 30 other doctors answered this advertisement and from this group, the DSN was born. We called it a network, meaning a loose alliance of doctors who had faced problems that in some way involved their mental health. We used the word 'troubled' to avoid the stigma of mental ill health and began our regular monthly meetings. Soames started the newsletter to keep those doctors who couldn't attend meetings informed about what the group discussed. We began to collect information about the resources available to doctors with mental health problems. This has developed into the DSL's Information Resource.

One of the strengths of the Doctors' Support Network and Doctors' Support Line is that contact between doctors is based not on position or job, rather contact is based on peer support. Over the last seven years there have been over a hundred meetings of the Doctors' Support Network.

The topics discussed at meetings are wide-ranging, although a number of themes consistently emerge. These include: the importance of our medical identity and the effect of mental illness on an individual's sense of self. Mental health problems go to the core of the individual. Mental health problems reflect beliefs, identity, capacity for work, energy and sensitivity to the environment and those around. They also reflect low self-esteem and uncertainty, in an environment where confidence and certainty are prerequisites of the job. Medicine is still more than a job, it is an identity and a way of life and way of being. When a doctor questions their ability to practise medicine, they are not only questioning their ability to earn a living, they are questioning who they are, their identity, and everything they believe about themselves. The meetings look at ways of restoring and reconnecting with an new identity. This may be medical but not necessarily. The meetings look at ways of developing and broadening that identity beyond medicine. The meetings look at ways of becoming more than the labels we give ourselves, more than the job title, the specialist label, more than the diagnostic label. We also value experiences outside medicine. The desire to help and connect with people defines who we are as people, not just who we are as a doctor. Medicine is demanding, and it can be a sink for all our energy and emotions, such that it is easy to believe that there is no life outside the hospital or clinic. It is important to remind ourselves that life has meaning outside medicine.

There is prejudice within the medical profession against mental illness, as a recent report by the Royal College of Psychiatrists[1] confirmed. Coping with the stigma of mental illness is not easy, not least because the very strength needed to stand up to the establishment and get the flexibility at work needed to continue working is the very strength that is eroded by illness. Meetings frequently debate the question of how much you should tell your prospective employers. The answer is usually the minimum necessary to achieve your goals. Furthermore, the emphasis is on putting one's experience of mental ill health in as positive a light as possible. Occupational Health combined with some hard-hitting government guidelines such as Improving Working Lives and the Disability Discrimination Act make it possible to get a fair deal from the NHS.

Other issues that are discussed in meetings include the role of occupational health and the punitive nature of the GMC. It has been the experience of almost all of the doctors in the network that facing the GMC for investigation of the state of their mental health has not been helpful. Yet until there is a change in the profession's attitude to mental illness, it will continue to be associated with conduct and performance and treated in a similar manner, with judicial proceedings rather than psychiatric help. Meetings also look at what to put in an application form when you have been off sick for a period of time and how to cover career gaps, and how to get retrained in a specialty. For doctors who are not working, contact with other doctors can be crucial in enabling them to feel part of medicine again. Although rehabilitation is not one of aims of the DSN, meeting other doctors has, in a number of cases, enabled some doctors to return to medicine. Other members of the Network have left medicine to contribute to society in other ways and to lead fulfilling lives that do not necessarily include doctoring.

The Doctors' Support Network has set up an email forum. This is a confidential group of 60 or more doctors which provides support, encouragement and advice for a range of personal and work-related problems. It is hard to believe that the people on the site are doctors, as the dialogue contradicts so much of what normally goes on between medics. People take time for each other and offer whatever help they can. Membership of the forum is open to members of the Doctors' Support Network.

The Doctors' Support Network makes demands on its committee and all who are involved in organising it. Perhaps one reason that mental health is generally the poor cousin is that people with poor mental health are generally short of energy. The energy they do have is needed to keep their head above water and hold down whatever job and family life they have. So the committee, whilst maintaining a clear management strategy for the organisation, needs to run by placing as few additional demands on its members as possible. As with any self-help group, it is important to make sure that no one is indispensable. From time to time, people appointed by the members to serve on the committee drop out of the committee because of their recurrent health problems and return when they are able to cope with it again. It is a tribute to the members of the committee and the Network as a whole that the organisation is still going from strength to strength after seven years. Those members who have set up local groups in their own areas deserve special thanks.

I have no doubt that the existence of the Doctors' Support Network and now the Doctors' Support Line has changed the climate in medicine. Seven years ago, more than one well known institution told us that our idea was very worthy but that mental ill health was not a significant problem amongst doctors. As we now have an organisation with more than 300 members, the mental health challenges faced by doctors are difficult to deny.

The challenge facing the Doctors' Support Network is to change the culture to one in which we are concerned with our own and each other's wellbeing. This will involve changing medical education to focus more on our own psychology and place more emphasis on health, both physical and mental. It will require that Trusts and PCTs show greater flexibility in training and rehabilitating doctors. We look to a future where we do not function as isolated individuals but as part of a caring professional community that accepts people for who they are and what they are capable of without discriminating against them on the basis of their health, gender or race. A culture that both supports doctors and helps them function to the best of their ability. Patients will ultimately benefit from being cared for by healthier, happier doctors who possess a greater awareness of themselves and those around them, including their patients.

if we could hug you and squeeze you tight
and get you through the long long nights
if we could keep your bad dreams away
so that you can live and fight another day
if we can keep your hopes alive
so that you do more than just plain old survive
if we can show you that there is someone out there
who will lend you an ear and may actually care.
if we can do this and more,
then depression will no longer darken your door

when you can use the past tense to talk about your pain and hurt
you will have forgotten about us in doctors' support network. . .

Anon

The Doctors' Support Network
Tel: 07071 223372
email: lizzie@dsn.org.uk
www.dsn.org.uk

Doctors' Support Line Tel: 0870 765 0001

Reference

1   Royal College of Psychiatrists (2001) *CR91. Mental Illness: stigmatisation and discrimination within the medical profession*. Royal College of Psychiatrists, London.

Summary

- DSN is a doctor-run national self-help group for doctors with mental health problems.
- Doctors' Support Line is a doctor-run helpline to support doctors troubled by personal home or work issues. It is also an information resource.
- DSN runs support groups around the country.
- The email network offers further opportunities for support and discussion.
- DSN hopes to challenge the prevailing culture of stigma towards mental illness.

Chapter 28

Resources

Heike Haffmans

General Medical Services

General practitioners

Doctors of all specialties and grades should be registered with a GP, GPs preferably not within their own surgery. Registration can be tricky in some areas, where many GP lists are full. Contact the local health authority to request a list of GPs and, if needed, allocation to a GP.

Doctors with frequent changes of job location, e.g. trainees, may prefer to stay registered with their 'home' GP. In this case it is advisable to register as a temporary resident with a local GP for the duration of their work placement away from home.

Different GP surgeries operate differently in how appointments are made. Generally it is possible to ask for double appointments when more time is needed for discussion. It is helpful to have seen/see your GP while well, as this gives your doctor a reference point. For any doctor looking after colleagues with chronic health problems, regular follow-ups and care plans are a good idea.

GPs should be the first point of contact for a doctor when medically unwell to access appropriate investigation and treatment. Self-investigation and self-treatment/prescribing is dangerous practice, potentially leading to misdiagnosis, delayed diagnosis and other complications to a doctor's health, as well as carrying the risk of professional consequences under the GMC regulations. Sick doctors should not take any medication other than those freely available to the public over the counter and those prescribed by a medical practitioner involved in their medical care.

A good relationship to a GP is crucial for successful medical management and continuity of care. Some GPs feel uncomfortable looking after colleagues and whether the therapeutic relationship works out is partly a matter of individual match. If there is any doubt about the suitability of an individual GP it is advisable to change GPs. It may be sufficient to change to a different partner within the same surgery.

Occupational Health services

The role of Occupational Health goes beyond the initial employment screening. Support should be offered to employees throughout their employment.

The employer has a responsibility in ensuring health and safety towards staff and Occupational Health has a role in monitoring this and implementing necessary changes not only for general health and safety issues, but also for any individual staff member. Occupational Health can negotiate adjustments to the workplace, including changing the work patterns to suit the need of the individual sick doctors and helping to plan the return to work after time off. In those respects an Occupational Health Physician can be a very useful ally to the sick doctor. In many Trusts staff can access further help, such as counselling, through Occupational Health.

A lot of mental and physical health problems are covered by the Disability Discrimination Act and Occupational Health can and should provide a link to the employer in a supportive manner. It is increasingly recognised that all doctors should have access to consultant-led Occupational Health services. Trusts need to ensure that such services are set up in a confidential manner. For more information:

Faculty of Occupational Medicine of the Royal College of Physicians
6 St Andrew's Place, Regent's Park, London NW1 4LB
Tel: 020 7317 5890
Fax: 020 7317 5899
email: fom@facoccmed.ac.uk
www.facoccmed.ac.uk

Professional services specialised in supporting doctors

It can be difficult for doctors to seek and access medical care within the 'normal' healthcare setting for various reasons. There is some concern over how privacy and confidentiality is maintained among other difficulties, when referred to local services, especially for doctors with psychiatric problems. Over the recent years there has been a growing recognition of doctors' health needs and their special situation as doctor patients. With this an increasing amount of regional and national support schemes which address doctors' welfare have become available.

Regional consultant-led counselling/psychotherapy self-referral services

These have been successfully set up in some regions of the UK in liaison with the deanery. Other regions may follow suit in the future. The services are accessible through self- referral and are strictly confidential with coded record systems, who do not report to other bodies.

The initial contact is made by phone. It may be necessary to leave your contact details on an answering service and wait a couple of days for someone to get back to you. For more information, make telephone contact.

House Concern in Newcastle upon Tyne (Northern Deanery)
Regional Department for Psychotherapy, Claremont House (off Framlington Place), Newcastle upon Tyne NE2 4AA
Tel: 0191 230 0043
Fax: 0191 227 5142

House Concern provides a clinical service for all doctors in the Northern Deanery and an educational service to all healthcare professionals. It provides a confidential, specialist, individual psychotherapy service, and enables access to longer term help if required. The service also includes educational seminars and lectures, workshops and group work focusing on issues of particular concern to doctors and other health professionals.

Take Time in Leeds (Yorkshire Deanery)
44 Clarendon Road, Leeds, LS2 9PJ
Tel: 0113 343 4642
Fax: 0113 343 4154
Take Time is a confidential counselling service for postgraduate doctors and dentists in training within the Yorkshire Deanery Leeds students counselling service and the NHS Specialist Psychotherapy Service in Leeds. Take Time offers two initial consultations to assess what is needed. These consultations may be enough in themselves or they may be followed by a period of brief counselling/ psychotherapy with Take Time staff. Access to longer term or other help if appropriate can be facilitated.

MedNet (London Deanery and Essex doctors)
Based at the Tavistock Clinic, London
Tel: 020 7447 3790
MedNet offers support to doctors working in the London and Essex region. The service offers six assessment consultations to assess what is needed and referral to longer term treatment if appropriate. The above telephone contact is manned for most of the day, otherwise an answer service is set up. Appointments can be usually made within two weeks.

Isis Centre (Oxford Deanery)
Little Clarendon Street, Oxford OX1 2HS
Tel: 01865 556648
The Isis Centre offers support to doctors in training working with a choice of CBT and psychodynamic psychotherapeutic treatment approaches. The service includes an initial assessment with subsequent discussion on needs and treatment options. The service is able to offer short-term intervention treatment support (average of six sessions) and can facilitate referral to other specialist services and long-term therapy when required.

BMA Doctors for Doctors Unit
Accessible to BMA members
www.bma.org link doctors' health and wellbeing.
The Doctors for Doctors Unit is committed to provide support for doctors in distress and difficulty by helping them make informed decisions about their health, working with them to gain insight, facilitating access to appropriate care and supporting them through this process.

The unit is developing its services and is only able to accept a limited number of self-referrals at present. The unit has produced a resource pack as a self-help tool to aid doctors in accessing appropriate help. The aim is to develop this site as an ongoing educational resource dealing with issues related to doctors' health.

The Sick Doctors Scheme, Association of Anaesthetists of GB and Ireland
Tel: 020 7631 1650
www.aagbi.org.uk
This service is available to anaesthetists of all grades and facilitates access to
psychological help though the scheme's advisor, who is an anaesthetist.[1]

BMA Counselling Service (24 hours)
Tel: 08459 200169
24-hour support confidential counselling helpline with immediate access to
trained counsellors. The service has been set up for BMA members and their
families, although someone making contact in acute crisis would not be likely to
be turned away immediately, just because of not being a member. The service can
point doctors to other sources of support.

'The Maudsley Sick Doctors Unit'
Part of South London and Maudsley Trust
Telephone enquiry line: 020 8776 4696
Referral to the service to: Prof. Anne Farmer, Lead Consultant
Affective Disorder Unit, Alexandra House 2, The Bethlehem Royal Hospital,
Monks Orchard Rd, Beckenham, Kent BR3 3BX
National in- and outpatient psychiatric service for doctors with affective disorders
and related dependencies.

   The Maudsley takes primary referrals for doctors nationwide (for other patients
referral is restricted to secondary and tertiary referrals). Referrals need to be made
via the sick doctors' GP and under the terms of service contract funding should be
provided by the referring local primary health authority. Under exceptional
circumstances self-referrals may be accepted. The initial referral is followed by
a first two-hour assessment. If indicated, hospital admission to the Affective
Disorder Unit in the Bethlehem Royal Hospital can be arranged electively or
(rarely) as an emergency. Alternatively, outpatient follow-up and access to
therapies can be arranged. The inpatient unit is a mixed unit, non-medical and
medical professional patients. The outpatient clinic is solely set up for doctors.

Self-help/peer support for doctors

The Doctors' Support Network
Tel: 0870 321 0642
email: info@dsn.org.uk
www.dsn.org.uk
DSN is a self-help group of medical professionals of all grades and specialties,
experiencing, recovering from or having recovered from mental and other health
problems, which has developed into a charitable organisation. Support is
provided by regular meetings in different parts of the country, monthly newsletter, email discussion group and helpful contacts throughout the country for
practical help for members. Membership is open to all members of the medical
profession who 'are suffering, are at risk of suffering and/or have recovered from
Mental Ill Health'. The primary aim of the group is to reduce the stigma and

isolation of mental health problems. Apart from providing peer support, the group can provide a wealth of information, helpful to all those who need help themselves or would like to help a colleague.

Doctors' Support Line
Tel: 0870 765 0001
(6pm–10pm Mon, Wed, Thu, Fri; 9am–2pm and 6pm–11pm Tue; 10am–10pm Sun)
www.doctorssupport.org
The DSL is an independent helpline, funded by the Department of Health for doctors in England. It was set up and is supported and administered by PriMHE in collaboration with the Doctors' Support Network.

All calls are answered by volunteer doctors from many different backgrounds offering a listening ear, mindful that callers are peers and not their patients. Please note that this is not a crisis service. For opening times and further info, ring in or visit the website.

The BMJ Careers Chronic Illness Matching Scheme
www.bma.org.uk/public/chill.nsf or www.bmj.careers.com
The chronic illness matching scheme provides the opportunity for doctors who have a chronic illness or disability to receive informal careers advice from another doctor and exchange experiences with doctors who have the same illness or careers.

The Sick Doctors Trust
Helpline: 0870 444 5163
www.sick-doctors-trust.co.uk
Confidential service for doctors set up by doctors to provide: early intervention in chemical dependency; training in its recognition; organise admissions when indicated; assistance with re-employment when required; support to their families.

The British Doctors' and Dentists' Group
Info via the secretary of the group: Tel: 01252 316976
Or can be accessed via the Medical Council on Alcoholism: Tel: 020 7487 4445
www.medicouncilalcol.demon.uk
Provides ongoing group support for doctors recovering from chemical dependency. It also welcomes students. Approximately 800 members and 16 local groups across the country. Monthly meetings.

International Doctors in Alcoholics Anonymous (IDAA)
www.idaa.org
IDAA is a group of approximately 4500 recovering healthcare professionals of doctorate level who help one another achieve and maintain sobriety from addictions.

The only requirement for membership is a desire to stay sober and off mood-altering drugs. The website provides information and resources for prospective and current members along with their family and friends – information on the organisation and links to other resources for recovery.

Career and work-related information and support for doctors and medical students

Postgraduate Dean/Associate Postgraduate Dean and Flexible Training Advisor and Royal College Tutors

Are able to help with career advice and/or part-time work when work abilities are affected by ill health or health is affected by work.

Some deaneries have special schemes to support and deal with ill doctors and/or underperforming doctors, e.g. Flexible Training Scheme for Doctors with Chronic Ill Health (Northern Deanery)[2] or Doctors in Difficulties (Mersey Deanery).[3]

UK Postgraduate Deaneries for Medicine and Dentistry

Eastern (Cambridge): www.easternregion.org.uk
Kent, Surrey and Sussex: www.kssdeanery.ac.uk
Leicestershire, Northampshire & Rutland: www.lnrdeanery.nhs.uk
Mersey (Liverpool): www.merseydeanery.ac.uk
Northern (Newcastle upon Tyne): www.pimd.co.uk
North-Western (Manchester): www.pgmd.man.ac.uk
Oxford (Oxford): www.oxford-pmgde.co.uk, www.oxdent.ac.uk
South-Western (Bristol): www.swndeanery.co.uk, www.dent.bris.ac.uk/dpg
North Thames (London): www.londondeanery.ac.uk
South Thames (London): www.londondeanery.ac.uk
South Yorkshire: www.sypgm.nhs
Trent: www.nottingham.ac.uk/mid-trent-deanery
Trent/Sheffield: www.pgde-trent.co.uk
Wessex (Winchester): www.wessex.org.uk
West Midlands (Birmingham): www.wmdeanery.org
Yorkshire (Leeds): www.yorkshiredeanery.com
Northern Ireland: www.nicpmde.com, www.nident.org.uk
Scotland: www.nes.scot.nhs.uk
Wales (Cardiff): www.postgrad-wales.org.uk, www.dentpostgradwales.ac.uk

Royal Colleges, societies and associations

The Royal Colleges will be able to advice on specific career paths, training requirements and training recognition (e.g. training recognition for individually set part-time training posts). There is a regional Royal College advisor for each specialty within a deanery, who can be contacted locally for career advice.

Membership of Royal Colleges is available to trainees training in the specialty. If a doctor is temporarily not working due to ill health and on low income, the college/society may look sympathetically on waiving the membership fee for a period of time, while continuing to offer the benefits.

Accident and emergency medicine
Faculty of Accident and Emergency Medicine, The Royal College of Surgeons of England
35/43 Lincoln's Inn Fields, London WC2A 3PN
Tel: 020 7405 7071

Anaesthetics
Association of Anaesthetists of Great Britain and Ireland (AAGBI)
21 Portland Place, London W1B 1PY
Tel: 020 7631 1650
Fax: 020 7631 4352
email: info@aagbi.org
www.aagbi.org.uk

Royal College of Anaesthetists
48–49 Russell Square, London WC1B 4JY
Tel: 020 7813 1900
www.rcoa.ac.uk

Intensive Care Society
9 Bedford Square, London WC1H 9HR
Tel: 020 7631 8890
www.ics.ac.uk

General practice
Royal College of General Practitioners
14 Prince Gate, London SW7 1PU
Tel: 020 7581 3232
www.rcgp.org.uk

The Joint Committee on Postgraduate Training and General Practice (JCPTGP)
1st Floor, 19 Buckingham Street, London WC2N 6EF
Tel: 020 7930 7228
Fax: 020 7930 7224
email: enquiry@jcptgp.org.uk
www.jcptgp.org.uk

Medicine
Royal College of Physicians (all specialties)
11 St Andrew Place, Regent's Park, London NW1 4IE
Tel: 020 7935 1174
www.rcplondon.ac.uk

Royal College of Physicians of Edinburgh
9 Queen Street, Edinburgh EH2 1JQ
Tel: 0131 225 7324
www.repe.ac.uk

Royal College of Physicians and Surgeons of Glasgow
232–242 St Vincent's Street, Glasgow G2 5RJ
Tel: 0141 221 6072
www.repsglasg.ac.uk

Royal College of Physicians of Ireland
6 Kildare Street, Dublin D2
Tel: 353 1 661 6677
www.repi.ie

Royal Society of Medicine
1 Wimpole Street, London W1G 0AE
Tel: 020 7290 2900
www.rsm.ac.uk

Obstetrics and gynaecology
Royal College of Obstetricians and Gynaecologists
27 Sussex Place, Regent's Park, London NW1 4RG
Tel: 020 7772 6200
www.repromed.net and www.rcog.org.uk

Faculty of Family Planning and Reproductive Healthcare
159 Cornwall Terrace, London NW1 4QP
Tel: 020 7935 7162

Occupational medicine
Faculty of Occupational Medicine of the Royal College of Physicians
6 St Andrew Place, Regent's Park, London NW1 4LB
Tel: 020 7317 5890
www.facoccmed.ac.uk

Ophthalmology
Royal College of Ophthalmologists
17 Cornwall Terrace, London NW1 4QW
Tel: 020 7935 0702
www.rcophth.ac.uk

Paediatrics
Royal College of Paediatrics and Child Health
50 Hallum Street, London WC1N 6DE
Tel: 020 7307 5600
www.rcpch.ac.uk

Pathology (with subspecialties)
Royal College of Pathologists
2 Carlton House Terrace, London SW1Y 5AF
Tel: 020 7451 6752
www.rcpath.org

Psychiatry (with subspecialties)
Royal College of Psychiatrists
17 Belgrave Square, London SW1X 8PG
Tel: 020 7235 2351
www.rcpsych.ac.uk

Public health
Faculty of Public Health Medicine
4 St Andrew's Place, London NW1 4LB
Tel: 020 7935 0243
www.fphm.org.uk

Radiology
Royal College of Radiologists
38 Portland Place, London W1N 4JQ
Tel: 020 7636 4432
www.rcr.ac.uk

Surgery
Royal College of Surgeons of Edinburgh
Nicolson Street, Edinburgh EH8 9DW
Tel: 0131 527 1600
www.rcsed.ac.uk

Royal College of Surgeons of England
35/43 Lincoln's Inn Fields, London WC2A 3PN
Tel: 020 7405 3474
www.rcseng.ac.uk

Royal College of Physicians and Surgeons of Glasgow
232–242 St Vincent's Street, Glasgow G2 5RJ
Tel: 0141 221 6072
www.rcpsglasg.ac.uk

Royal College of Surgeons in Ireland
St Stephen's Green, Dublin D2
Tel: 00 353 1 412 2100
www.rcsi.ie

General
General Medical Council (GMC)
178 Great Portland Street, London W1N 6JE
General enquiries: Tel: 020 7580 7642
www.gmc-uk.org
Doctors' fitness to practise guide/advice: Tel: 0845 357 0022
email: practise@gmc-uk.org
GMC health procedures: Tel: 020 7915 3580

email: health@gmc-uk.org
GMC performance procedures: Tel: 020 7915 3667
email: performance@gmc-uk.org

British Medical Association (BMA)
BMA House, Tavistock Square, London WC1H 9JR
Tel: 020 7387 4499
Fax: 020 7383 6400
email: info.web@bma.org.uk
www.bma.org.uk
BMA local offices: www.bma.org.uk/localoffices
The BMA is an independent trade union representing doctors in all branches of medicine all over the UK and includes members overseas. It offers a range of services to its members and can provide helpful advice and support in relation to employment issues.

Medical Forum
24 Woodlands, Overton, Hants RG25 3HN
Tel: 0705 007 7171 or 07000 790173
Fax: 0705 007 7272
www.medicalforum.com
Medical Forum is a private 'career management facility', providing an independent personal career review, assessment and advice service. It offers web-based support: newsletter; 'ask career mentor'; e-courses on career handling skills such as study, stress, saying no, defining success, and change; training materials and publications; psychometric testing; tailored, innovative training workshops such as career guidance essentials, and avoiding the career plateau; distance learning 'career review'; one-to-one 'Personal Career Programmes'; a membership club for those who have successfully completed the programmes; and 'career tutor' membership for those providing career support to others.

Costs depend on extent of assessment. Deaneries may in some cases be amenable to provide funding for some of those services. Workbook free for DSN members.

NHS Professionals Services
Tel: 0845 60 60 345
email: medical@nhsprofessionals.nhs.uk
www.nhs.uk/nhsprofessionals
NHS Professionals Services can help doctors with access to a range of services. These include:

- long and short-term locum placements through their not-for profit locum service
- assistance with appraisal and revalidation programme
- Training Credit Scheme
- Flexible Career Scheme (*see* part-time work opportunities, opposite)
- New Consultants Entry Scheme
- facilitation of recruitment of international doctors by supporting them.

There are numerous regional offices.

Part-time work opportunities

Flexible Career Scheme
www.nhscareer.nhs.uk
The Flexible Career Scheme is administered by NHS Professionals on behalf of the Department of Health and empowers doctors to plan their own career. It is *available to all doctors*, including GPs, and is particularly designed for those who:

- wish to move temporarily into a limited hours role
- would like a career break, but wish to keep in touch with the profession
- are retired, semi-retired or nearing retirement from the NHS and wish to work in reduced capacity
- are currently not working but wish to return to practice and require a period of supervision.

The posts are supernumerary and limited to a maximum of five sessions with no on-call commitment and no training recognition. The contract and work time-table can be negotiated taking into account individual circumstances (for example, a doctor returning from a career break due to ill health may start work as little as one hour per day and gradually build up the workload over a period of time). The posts are time limited to a maximum of two years with possible one year extension. Application for these posts involves negotiations with the local Trust, which will employ the doctor. Liaison with the Associate Postgraduate Dean may also be required.

Flexible Training
Funding for Flexible Training is administered through the Associate Postgraduate Dean of the individual region. Due to funding shortage *only doctors with 'good reasons'* (e.g. illness and family commitments) *for needing part-time training are eligible for these posts*. These posts require a minimum of 50% of full-time work commitment including on-call commitments. Some post are set up as super-numerary posts but increasingly these posts become part of jobshare-type arrangements administered by the deanery. Application is competitive and generally involves securing an offer for a regular post prior to applying for Flexible Training. There might be exceptions under certain circumstances. For details on how to apply contact the Associate Postgraduate Dean of the region.

Flexible Training Scheme for doctors with disabilities/chronic ill health
This scheme was set up in the Northern Deanery by the Flexible Training Advisor together with a consultant in Occupational Health. It has been very successful in helping trainees who cannot work full-time and often not in a fixed part-time post to continue and complete their training by working in supernumerary part-time posts. Regular reviews with the Occupational Health Consultant take place for any trainee on the programme and alterations to work pattern and hours are made depending on need.

Jobshare
Jobshare is an alternative way of working part-time for doctors in training and non-training grades. Setting up a jobshare post requires some planning. The PGI

can be helpful in setting up such posts for trainees. The BMA can help with employment issues.

BMJ Careers
www.bmjcareers.com

BMJ Career Focus
Editor: Graham Easton
Tel: 020 7383 6125
email: careerfocus@bmj.com
The BMJ Career Focus is part of the weekly BMJ and addresses a great variety of career and personal development issues. It is a rich and well designed source of information for any doctor, in particular those who are unable or unwilling to follow the streamline career path.

BMJ Career Fair
A yearly event organised by the BMJ. Held in recent years in November in London. The event offers a range of workshops, talks and stands relating to a great variety of medical career issues and professional development. It is free for BMA members.

If attendance of such an event is important for the stage of career you find yourself at, you might be able to negotiate funding for it as study leave from your Postgraduate Institute.

Access to Work Scheme
The Access to Work is a programme run by the Department for Work and Pensions and administered through the Jobcentre Plus. It provides support to disabled people to help them overcome work-related obstacles resulting from their disability if this is likely to last longer than 12 months. Any person who becomes disabled under the criteria of the Disability Discrimination Act is eligible to apply. Following application a needs assessment is made by an independent assessor from Access to Work, who then prepares a report outlining the requirements to meet the disabled person's needs and the estimated cost.

Help can include aids for communication, special equipment, alterations to the premises, support worker, assistance with communication and travel.

The employer purchases the equipment and claims the expenses back from the Access to Work Scheme. It is helpful to involve Occupational Health in the application process.

For further information and links to contacts for local Disability Service/Access to Work Teams, visit www.jobcentreplus.gov.uk

Healthy Return to Work
Freephone: 0800 052 1012
email: info@healthyreturn.org
www.healthyreturn.org
Healthy Return is a two-year pilot study started on 1 April 2003. This main aim of the project is to test what, if any, benefit the provision of additional services has on helping people back to health and work. There are six centres in the UK:

Greater Glasgow, West Kent, Birmingham, Teesside, Tyneside and Sheffield. As a randomised controlled trial, all eligible volunteers are allocated in one of four pathways: healthcare, workplace care, combined health and work care and control group.

Association of Disabled Professionals

BCM ADP, London WC1N 3XX
Tel: 01204 431638
Fax: 01204 431638
email: adp.admin@ntlworld.com
www.adp.org.uk

Disability Rights Commission

DRC Helpline, FREEPOST MID02164, Stratford upon Avon, CV37 9BR
Helpline: Tel: 08457 622 633; Textphone: 08457 622 644
(You can speak to an operator at any time between 8am and 8pm, Monday to Friday)
Fax: 08457 778 878
www.drc-gb.org
Gives advice on the Disability Discrimination Act, information material for organisations and individuals.

Skill: National Bureau for Students with Disabilities

Head Office: Chapter House, 18–20 Crucifix Lane, London SE1 3JW
Tel/Minicom: 020 7450 0620
Fax: 020 7450 0650
email: skill@skill.org.uk
Information service: Freephone 0800 328 5050 and 020 7657 2337 (open Tuesdays 11.30am to 1.30pm and Thursdays 1.30–3.30pm)
Minicom: 0800 068 2422
email: info@skill.org.uk
www.skill.org.uk

Skill in Northern Ireland

Unit 2, Jennymount Court, North Derby Street, Belfast BT15 3HN
Tel/Minicom: 0289 028 7000
Fax: 0289 028 7002
email: admin@skillni.org.uk

Skill in Scotland

Norton Park, 57 Albion Road, Edinburgh EH7 5QY
Tel/Minicom: 0131 475 2348
Fax: 0131 475 2397
email: admin@skillscotland.org.uk

Health and Safety at Work

Zero Tolerance Campaign
NHS Executive HQ, Quarry House, Quarry Hill, Leeds LSE 7UE
Tel: 08701 555 455
www.nhs.uk/zerotolerance
Addresses issues and provides support in relation to harassment and violence towards NHS staff in the workplace.

Health and Safety Executive (HSE) (local offices across the UK)
London Information Centre (9am–5pm, Monday–Friday): Health and Safety Executive, Rose Court, 2 Southwark Bridge, London SE1 9HS
Bootle Information Centre (9am–5pm, Monday–Friday): Health and Safety Executive, Magdalen House, Trinity Road, Bootle, Merseyside L20 3QZ
Telephone info-line: 0870 154 5500 (8am–6pm, Monday–Friday)
email: hseinformationservice@natbrit.com
www.hse.gov.uk
Provides rapid access to HSE's wealth of health and safety information, and access to expert advice and guidance.

Employment Medical Advisory Service (EMAS), Health and Safety Executive
The Employment Medical Advisory Service is part of FOD (Field Operations Directorate of the HSE). It supports all HSE's front-line activities and provides Occupational Health advice direct to employers and employees. EMAS has offices throughout the country that are staffed by doctors and nurses with Occupational Health qualifications. EMAS provides free advice and support to employers and employees regarding work-related medical problems, including mental health problems. Contact through the HSE local offices.

Worker Webpage
www.hse.gov.uk/workers
Health and Safety Executive worker's webpage provides information on rights and responsibilities, accidents, whistle blowing

NHS Health Development Agency (HDA)
Health Development Agency, Holborn Gate, 330 High Holborn, London WC1V 7BA
Tel: 020 7430 0850
Fax: 020 7061 3390
www.hda-online.org.uk
The HAD is the national authority on what works to improve people's health and to reduce health inequalities. The HAD offers a range of expertise on mental health and wellbeing and various aspects of workplace health and wellbeing.

The International Stress Management Association
PO Box 348, Waltham Cross EN8 8ZL
Tel: 07000 780430
email: stress@isma.org.uk
www.isma.org.uk

The International Stress Management Association is a charity that aims to promote sound knowledge and best practice in the prevention and reduction of human stress. It sets professional standards for the benefit of individuals and organisations using the service and of its members.

Financial and legal issues, welfare and practical support

Every doctor is well advised to take out some private insurance policy at the earliest stage possible, which will cover for loss of income due to sickness and early retirement. Where there is no private support the following can help.

Royal Medical Benevolent Fund
24 King's Rd, Wimbledon, London SW19 8QN
Tel: 020 8540 9194
Fax: 020 8542 0494
email: info@rmbf.org
www.rmbf.org
The Royal Medical Benevolent Fund is a registered charity, which offers financial help to any member of the medical profession registered with the GMC and resident in the UK and their dependants, who is in financial need with little in the way of income or savings and who might already receive any relevant state benefit.

Help includes regular financial support, interest-free loans, one-off grants and information and advice from experienced caseworkers.

In some cases it may already help sufficiently to go through the structured process of advice to find a way to manage finances better.

Following making contact an assessment of the financial situation, i.e. income versus spending, is made. Applications for support are treated in confidence. Advice on eligibility for other benefits can also be given. A decision about support is made according to priorities.

BMA Charities
The BMA Charities Trust Fund, BMA House, Tavistock Square, London, WC1H 9JP
Tel: 020 7383 6334
www.bma.org.uk
The BMA Charities Trust Fund receives donations and investment income, which it uses to make major grants to other charities whose purpose is the relief of the need of doctors and their dependants. *Support is available independent of BMA membership.*

The Hastings Benevolent Fund:[4] Provides short-term financial assistance to doctors and/or their dependants. Support is also given to refugee doctors with PLAB exam fees and GMG registration fees.

BMA Medical Education Trust:[4] Supports medical students in financial need, in particular the mature students studying medicine as second degree, with grants.

The Dain Fund:[4] Assists with the educational expenses of doctors' children (school and higher education) when a family crisis threatens the continuity of that education.

The Cameron Fund
Tavistock House North, Tavistock Square, London WC1H 9HR
Tel: 020 7388 0796
The Cameron Fund is a charity which supports GPs and their dependants in times of poverty, hardship and distress with financial support in a similar way to the above charities. Applications are treated in strictest confidence.

National Health Pension Agency
Tel: 01253 774 774 (8.30–17.00 Monday–Thursday, 8.30–16.30 Friday)
www.nhspa.gov.uk
Sick/Disabled doctors may be entitled to a pension under the NHS Pension Scheme, if illness is work-related. It is advisable to get a professional pension advisor to help you with your claim. BMA members can get help via the BMA pension advisor.

Department for Work and Pensions (DWP)
Benefits enquiry line: 0800 88 22 00
Textphone: 0800 243 355
www.dwp.gov.uk
This website gives information on a wide range of services and benefits.

Sick/Disabled doctors may be entitled to a number of benefits such as Incapacity Benefit, Income Support, Council Tax Benefit, Industrial Injury Benefit, Disability Living Allowance etc. It is strongly advisable to engage the help of a Citizens Advice Bureau advisor/welfare rights officer when making claims.

www.direct.gov.uk
A helpful website, providing a wide range of public service information, including giving advice on money matters with helpful links.

Citizens Advice Bureau
See local phone directory for telephone number of nearest office.

Provides a range of free and confidential services. Will be able to advise on benefit entitlements and other services available in the community. A Citizens Advice Bureau advisor is an invaluable help when it comes to filling in benefit forms and dealing with the DWP. Offers legal advice and support in disputes with the DWP benefit decisions.
www.citizensadvice.org.uk
Gives directory of all offices and advice by email.
www.adviceguide.org.uk
Advice guide website.

Citizen Advice Scotland
www.cas.org.uk

Social services
Able to provide practical support and care. Also point of contact to obtain disabled car badge. For contact consult local telephone directory and/or ask GP.

Local MPs

If you find you get unfair treatment by a government or related department, such as the DWP, it is a good idea to contact and inform your local MP. He/she is in a position to raise your concerns at higher levels and support you.

MDU

MDU Services Limited, 230 Blackfriars Road, London SE1 8PJ
Tel: 020 7202 1500
Fax: 020 7202 1696
General enquiries: email: mdu@the-mdu.com
www.the-mdu.com
Membership Helpline: 0800 716 376
Advisory services, claims, risk management: Freephone 0800 716 646 (24 hours)
email: advisory@the-mdu.com
MDU is a medical defence union who offers a range of advisory and support services in risk management and legal issues and supports members with legal assistance and indemnity cover for compensation claims.

Shelter

Admin: 88 Old Street, London EC1V 9HU
Tel: 020 7505 4699
email: info@shelter.co.uk
Helpline: 0808 800 4444 (24 hour)
www.shelter.org.uk
General advice on housing problems for England, Scotland, Wales and Northern Ireland.

Support for specific groups among doctors

Doctors from outside the UK

International Department (includes Refugee Doctor Liaison Group)
BMA House, Tavistock Square, London WC1H 9JP
Tel: 020 7383 6133/6793
Fax: 020 7383 6644
email: internationalinfo.web@bma.org.uk
www.bma.org.uk/international

NHS Professionals
4th Floor, Don Valley House, Savile Street East, Sheffield S4 7UQ
Tel: 0845 120 3164
Fax: 0114 275 8008
Provides an induction course for non-UK graduated doctors undertaking their first appointment in the NHS on behalf of the deaneries. Free of charge.

Homosexual doctors

Gay and Lesbian Association of Doctors and Dentists (GLADD)
BM Box 5606, London WC1N 3XX
Tel: 0870 765 5606 (national rates)
email: secretary@gladd.org.uk
www.gladd.org.uk

Women

Medical Women's Federation
Tavistock House North, Tavistock Square, London WC1H 9HX
Tel: 020 7387 7765
Fax: 020 7388 9216
email: mwf@btconnect.com
www.medicalwomensfederation.co.uk

Women in Surgical Training (WIST)
The Royal College of Surgeons in England
35/43 Lincoln's Inn Fields, London WC2A 3PE
Tel: 020 7405 3474
www.rcseng.ac.uk/surgical/trainees/wist/
WIST is a national organisation working to promote surgery as a career for women and to enable women who have chosen a career in surgery to realise their professional goals.

Further helpful contacts

The following contacts are national self-help, non-statutory and voluntary organisations, which are accessible to the general public and can be equally valuable to doctors. Many of these agencies have offices and networks of support groups across the country. Some may only provide support through membership. There are many more such agencies providing information and support for people in distress through illness or other circumstances and their carers. It is beyond the scope of this chapter to be all-inclusive and only a selection of those services is listed.

General health

Doctor Patient Partnership (DPP)
Tavistock House, Tavistock Square, London WC1 9JP
Tel: 020 7383 6715
Fax: 020 7383 6966
email: dpp@bma.org.uk
www.dpp.org.uk
The DPP is a charitable organisation, providing patient education material to both healthcare professionals and the general public. The aim is to encourage better communication between healthcare professionals and patients, promote the responsible use of the NHS and offer practical advice on medication.

The website offers a wealth of information, including information leaflets and book references, as well as references to other Patient Associations.

General mental health

African Caribbean Mental Health Association (ACMHA)
Suites 34 & 37, 49 Efra Road, London SW2 1BZ
Tel: 020 7737 3603
Community Mental Health Centre that provides a range of care services for the black community.

C.A.U.S.E. for Mental Health
1st Floor, Glendinning House, 6 Murray Street, Belfast BT1 6DN
Office Tel: 028 9023 8284
Fax: 028 9024 3838
Helpline: 0845 603 0291
email: info@cause.org.uk
www.cause.org.uk

Mental Health Foundation
UK office: 7th Floor, 83 Victoria Street, London SW1H 0HW
Tel: 020 7802 0300
Fax: 020 7802 0301
email: mhf@mhf.org.uk
Scotland office: 5th Floor, Merchants House, 30 George Square, Glasgow G2 1EG
Tel: 0141 572 0125
Fax: 0141 572 0246
email: scotland@mhf.org.uk
www.mentalhealth.org.uk
Free leaflets about mental illness and learning disabilities for the general public.

MIND
Granta House, 15–19 Broadway, Stratford, London E15 4BQ
Office: Tel: 020 8519 2122
Fax: 020 8522 1725
email: contact@mind.org.uk
MINDinfoLINE: 0845 766 0163
email: info@mind.org.uk
www.mind.org.uk
Information service for matters relating to mental health.
Mind Cymru
3rd Floor, Quebec House, Castlebridge, 5–19 Cowbridge Road East, Cardiff CF11 9AB
Tel: 029 2039 5123
Fax: 029 2034 6585
Rural Minds
c/o South Staffs CVS, 1 Stafford Street, Brewood, Staffs ST19 9DX
Tel: 024 7641 4366
Fax: 024 7641 4369
email: ruralminds@ruralnet.org.uk

Northern Ireland Association for Mental Health (NIAMH)
Central Office, 80 University Street, Belfast BT7 1HE
Tel: 028 9032 8474
www.niamh.co.uk
Provides services in the community for people with mental needs.

Rethink (formerly the National Schizophrenia Fellowship) (local groups)
28 Castle Street, Kingston-upon-Thames, Surrey KT1 1SS
General enquiries: Tel: 0845 456 0455
email: info@rethink.org
Advice line: 020 8974 6814 (10am–3pm, Monday–Friday)
email: advice@rethink.org
www.rethink.org
Works to help everyone affected by severe mental illness, including schizophrenia, to recover a better quality of life. More than 300 services in England, Wales and Northern Ireland provided, including home treatment, nursing care, carers' support, helplines and advocacy.

SANELine
Helpline: 08457 678 000 (12 noon–2 am daily)
www.sane.org.uk
Helpline offering information and advice on all aspects of mental health for those experiencing illness or their families or friends.
SANE in London: 1st Floor Cityside House, 40 Adler Street, London E1 1EE
Tel: 020 7375 1002
Fax: 020 7375 2162
email: london@sane.org.uk
SANE in Bristol: Units 1 & 2, The Greenway Centre, Doncaster Road, Southmead, Bristol BS10 5PY
Tel: 0117 950 2140
Fax: 0117 950 2150
email: bristol@sane.org.uk
SANE in Macclesfield: 1 Queen Victoria Street, Macclesfield SK11 6LP
Tel: 01625 429 050
Fax: 01625 424 975
email: macclesfield@sane.org.uk

Scottish Association for Mental Health
Cumbrae House, 15 Carlton Court, Glasgow G5 9JP
Tel: 0141 568 7000
Fax: 0141 568 7001
email: enquiries@samh.org.uk
www.samh.org.uk

Someone To Talk To
PO Box 245, St Albans, Hertfordshire AL3 5YW
email: advice@someonetotalkto.co.uk
www.someonetotalkto.co.uk

Someone To Talk To offers free advice and support and confidential counselling by qualified therapists and counsellors on issues such as relationship difficulties and breakdowns, stress, depression, anxiety and other mental health worries, via email, phone and post.

Specific problems

Alcohol misuse

Al-Anon Family Groups UK and Eire (local groups)
England: 61 Great Dover Street, London SE1 4YF
Tel: 020 7403 0888
www.al-anon.org
EIRE: Al-Anon Info Centre, Room 5, Chapel Street, Dublin 1, Eire
Tel: 353 1873 2699
Northern Ireland: Al-Anon Info Centre, Peace House, 224 Lisburn Road, Belfast BT9 6GE
Tel: 028 9068 2368
Scotland: Al-Anon Info Centre, Mansfield Park Unit 6, 22 Mansfield Street, Partick, Glasgow G11 5QP
Tel: 0141 339 8884
Understanding and support for families and friends of alcoholics, whether still drinking or not.

Alateen
Helpline: 020 7403 0888 (10am–10pm, daily)
www.al-anon.alateen.org
For young people aged 12–20 affected by others' drinking.

Alcohol Advisory Service
309 Grays Inn Road, London WC1X 8QF
Tel: 020 7530 5900
(Similar services are available in other parts of the country.)

Alcoholics Anonymous (local groups)
General Service Office, PO Box 1, Stonebow House, Stonebow, York YO1 7NJ
Administration: Tel: 01904 644 026
Helpline: 0845 7697555
London helpline: 020 7833 0022 (10am–10pm daily)
email: aanewcomer@runbox.com
www.alcoholics-anonymous.org.uk
Confidential helpline, email and support groups for women and men trying to achieve and maintain sobriety and help other alcoholics to get sober.

Alcohol Concern
Waterbridge House, 32–36 Loman Street, London SE1 0EE
Admin: Tel: 020 7928 7377
Fax: 020 7928 4644
email: contact@alcoholconcern.org.uk

Helpline (through Drinkline National Alcohol Helpline): 0800 917 8282 (24 hours)
www.alcoholconcern.org.uk
Alcohol Concern is the national agency on alcohol misuse. It supplies information on and any details on local services.

Drinkline National Alcohol Helpline
Freepost, PO Box 4000, Glasgow G3 8XX
Helpline: 0800 917 8282
Asian line (Hindu, Urdu, Gujarati, Punjabi): 0990 133 480 (1pm–8pm, Monday)
Confidential alcohol counselling and information service.

Down Your Drink
www.downyourdrink.org.uk
Online programme to help reduce and control drinking.

Medical Council on Alcoholism
3 St Andrew's Place, Regent's Park, London NW1 4LB
Tel: 020 7487 4445
Fax: 020 7935 4479
email: mca@medicouncilalcol.demon.co.uk
www.medicouncilalcol.demon.co.uk
Medical professionals, interested in alcohol, not simply to pursue an academic or personal consuming interest though, but 'for the benefit of the community to provide an organization of registered medical practitioners with a view to co-ordination of effort, the better understanding of alcoholism and its prevention and the treatment and after-care of alcoholics'. Network of regional advisors for information and education.

National Association for Children of Alcoholics
PO Box 64, Fishponds, Bristol BS16 2UH
Admin: Tel: 0117 924 8005
Fax: 0117 942 2928
email: admin@nacoa.org.uk
Helpline: 0800 358 3456 (10am–7pm, Monday, Tuesday, Thursday, Friday; 10am–9pm Wednesday; 10am–3pm Saturday)
email: help@nacoa.org.uk
www.nacoa.org.uk
Provides support and information to children of alcoholics.

North Ireland Community Addiction Service (additional local branches)
40 Elmwood Avenue, Belfast BT9 6AZ
Tel: 028 9066 4434 (8.45am–5pm Monday–Thursday, 8.45am–1pm Fridays)
Fax: 028 9066 4090
email:nicas@dial.pipex.com

Anxiety, obsessive-compulsive disorder, panic and phobias
The International Stress Management Association (ISMA) UK
PO Box 348, Waltham Cross EN8 8ZL
Tel: 07000 780 430
email: stress@isma.org.uk
www.isma.org.uk
Promotes knowledge and best practice in the prevention and management of acute stress.

First Steps to Freedom (local groups)
1 Taylor Close, Kenilworth, Warwickshire CV8 2LW
Office: Tel: 01926 864 473
Fax: 0870 164 0567
Helpline: 0845 120 2916
email: info@firststeps.demon.co.uk
www.first-steps.org
Self-help groups.

No Panic (local groups)
23 Brands Farm Way, Telford TF3 2JQ
Office: Tel: 01952 590 005
Fax: 01952 270962
email: ceo@nopanic.org.uk
Helpline: 0808 808 0545 (10am–10pm daily and a taped crisis message through the night)
www.nopanic.org.uk

OCD Action
Aberdeen Centre, 22–24 Highbury Grove, London N5 2EA
Tel: 020 7226 4000
Fax: 020 7288 0828
email: info@ocdaction.org.uk
www.ocdaction.org.uk
Information, advice and support for people with obsessive-compulsive disorder and related disorders such as body dysmorphic disorder and trichotillomania.

Social Anxiety UK (local groups)
email: contact@social-anxiety.org.uk
www.social-anxiety.org.uk
Information and support for sufferers of social anxiety and related problems. Chat room and local meetings across the UK.

Stresswatch Scotland (local groups)
Helpline: 01563 574144 (10am–10pm daily, panic advice tape recording out of these hours)
Advice, information, materials on panic, anxiety, stress, phobias.

Triumph over Phobia (TOP UK) (local groups)
PO Box 344, Bristol BS34 8ZR
Tel: 0845 600 9601
email: triumphoverphobia@compuserve.com
www.triumphoverphobia.com
Structured self-help groups for sufferers from phobias or obsessive-compulsive disorder. Produces self-help materials.

Bipolar disorder
The Manic Depression Fellowship (MDF)
England: Castle Works, 21 St George's Road, London SE1 6ES
Office: Tel: 020 7793 2600
Fax: 020 7793 2639
Infoline: 0845 634 0540
Email: mdf@mdf.org.uk (information); smt@mdf.org.uk (self-management); groups@mdf.org.uk (self-help groups)
www.mdf.org.uk
Wales: 1 Palmyra Place, Newport, South Wales, NP20 4EJ
Helpline: 08456 340 080
email: info@mdfwales.org.uk
www.mdfwales.org.uk
Advice, support, local self-help groups and publications list for people with a manic depressive illness.

MDF Scotland
1016 Abbey Mill Business Park, Seedhill Road, Paisley PA1 1TJ
Tel: 0141 560 2050
email: info@mdfscotland.co.uk
www.mdfscotland.co.uk
Separate charity to MDF England and Wales, providing similar service in Scotland.

Carers
Carers UK
UK Office: 20–25 Glasshouse Yard, London EC1A 4JT
Tel: 020 7490 8818
Fax: 020 7490 8824
email: info@ukcarers.org.uk
www.carersonline.org.uk
Helpline: 0808 808 7777 (10am–12noon and 2–4pm, Monday–Friday)
North of England: 23 New Mount Street, Manchester M4 4DE
Tel: 0161 953 4233
Fax: 0161 953 4092
Northern Ireland: 58 Howard Street, Belfast BT1 6PJ
Tel: 028 9043 9843
Fax: 028 9043 9299
email: info@carersni.demon.co.uk

Scotland: 91 Mitchell Street, Glasgow G1 3LN
Tel: 0141 221 9141
Fax: 0141 221 9140
email: information@carerscotland.org
Wales: River House, Ynysbridge Court, Gwaelod y Garth, Cardiff CF15 9SS
Tel: 029 2081 1370
Fax: 029 2081 1575
email: info@carerswales.demon.co.uk
Formerly the National Carers Association. Provides information and advice on all aspects of care for both carers and professionals.

Crossroads Association (local groups)
10 Regent Place, Rugby CV21 2PN
Tel: 0845 450 0350
Fax: 0845 450 0350
email: communications@crossroads.org.uk
www.crossroads.org.uk
There are regional centres throughout the UK, providing practical support and help for carers, including respite care, day centres, befriending and night care. There is a scheme for young carers also.

Debt
National Debtline
The Arch, 48–52 Floodgate Street, Birmingham B5 5SL
Freephone: 0808 808 4000
Fax: 0121 703 6940
www.nationaldebtline.co.uk

Depression
Aware Defeat Depression Ltd. (local groups)
10 Clarendon Street, Derry, Co Londonderry BT48 7DA
Tel: 02871 260 602
Fax: 02871 309 229
email: info@aware-ni.org
www.aware-ni.org
Provides information leaflets, lectures and runs support groups for sufferers and relatives.

Campaign Against Living Miserably (CALM)
Helpline: 0800 585 858
Helpline for 15 to 24-year-old men at the onset of depression, to give advice, guidance, referrals and counselling.

Depression Alliance (local groups)
Main tel: 0845 123 2320 (will provide access to regional contacts)
England: 35 Westminster Bridge Road, London SE1 7JB
Wales: 11 Plas Melin, Westbourne Rd, Whitchurch, Cardiff CF14 2BT
Tel: 029 2069 2891
email: wales@depressionaliance.org

Scotland: 3 Grosvenor Gardens, Edinburgh EH12 5JU
Tel: 0131 467 3050
Fax: 0131 467 7701
www.depressionalliance.org
Provides information and self-help groups.

Depressives Anonymous
36 Chestnut Avenue, Beverly, East Yorkshire HU17 9QU
Tel: 01482 860619
An organisation run as a source of support to sufferers. Can put caller in contact with local groups.

SAD (Seasonal Affective Disorder) Association
PO Box 989, Steyning BN44 3HG
Tel: 01903 814 942
www.sada.org.uk
Information about seasonal affective disorder (SAD). Offers advice and support to members.

Association for Postnatal Illness
145 Dawes Road, London SW6 7EB
Helpline: 020 7386 0868
Fax: 020 7386 8885
email: info@apni.org
www.apni.org
Information on postnatal depression, and will put affected mothers in touch with others who have had similar experiences.

Disability issues
Ability on line
www.abilityonline.net
Disability website providing a wide range of information and links on disability issues, including benefits.

Association of Disabled Professionals
BCM ADP, London WC1N 3XX
Tel: 01204 431638
Fax: 01204 431638
email: adp.admin@ntlworld.com
www.adp.org.uk

Disability Rights Commission
DRC Helpline, FREEPOST MID02164, Stratford upon Avon, CV37 9BR
Helpline: Tel: 08457 622 633; Textphone: 08457 622 644
(You can speak to an operator at any time between 8am and 8pm, Mon to Fri)
Fax: 08457 778 878
Gives advice on the Disability Discrimination Act, information material for organisations and individuals.

DisabledGo
Unit 4 Brick Knoll Park, Ashley Rd Industrial Estate, St Albans, Hertfordshire
AL1 5UG
email: info@disabledgo.info
www.disabledgoinfo.com
Internet service providing information for disabled people.

Domestic violence
Domestic Violence Unit or Community Safety Unit
Contact your local Police Force for details.

Everyman Project
40 Stockwell Road, Stockwell, London SW9 9ES
Tel: 020 7737 6747
Fax: 020 7737 6747
www.changeweb.org.uk/new_page_22.htm
Counselling, support and advice to men who are violent or concerned about their
violence, and anyone affected by that violence.

Kiran: Asian Women's Aid
Tel: 020 8558 1986
Fax: 020 8532 8260
email: kiranawa@btopenworld.com
Advice, support, refuge for Asian women, and women from other cultures (e.g.
Turkey, Iran, Morocco and Malaysia).

Refuge
2/8 Maltravers Street, London WC2R 3EE
Office: Tel: 020 7395 7700
email: info@refuge.org.uk
24-hour National Domestic Violence Helpline: 0808 2000 247
www.refuge.org.uk
Offers support, information and referrals. Runs own refuges.

Relate
Local branches across the UK including NI, the Isle of Man, Channel Islands and
Scotland. Contact details for individual branches listed on website.
Helpline/Booking line: 08451 304 016
www.relate.org.uk
Relate offers advice, relationship counselling, sex therapy, workshops, medita-
tion, support by face-to-face consultations, by phone and through information on
the website.

Women's Aid Federation
PO Box 391, Bristol BS99 7WS
Freephone National Domestic Violence 24-hour Helpline: 0808 2000 247
Run in partnership with refuge.

email: helpline@womensaid.org.uk
www.womensaid.org.uk
Wide range of support and advice services, information and refuge referrals for
women and their children experiencing domestic violence.

Worst Kept Secret
PO Box 182, Liverpool L69 2SW
Tel: 0151 227 5808
Helpline: 0800 028 3398
email: wks@btconnect.com
www.domesticviolenceprevention.com
Information, support and prevention relating to domestic violence.

Drug misuse
ADFAM National
Waterbridge House, 32–36 Loman Street, London SE1 0EH
Tel: 020 7928 8923
Fax: 020 7928 8898
email: admin@adfam.org.uk
www.adfam.org.uk
Confidential support and information for families and friends of drug users.

CITA (Council for Involuntary Tranquilliser Addiction)
CITA, The JDI Centre, 3–11 Mersey View, Waterloo, Liverpool L22 5NG
Office: Tel: 0151 474 9626
Helpline: 0151 932 0102 (10am–1pm, Monday–Friday: emergency weekend
number available)
Related website: www.benzo.org.uk
Offers advice on withdrawing from tranquillisers and help with anxiety and
depression.

DrugScope
32–36 Loman Street, London SE1 0EE
Tel: 020 7928 1211
Fax: 020 7928 1771
email: info@drugscope.org.uk
www.drugscope.org.uk
UK's leading independent centre of expertise on drugs.

Families Anonymous (local groups)
The Doddington and Rollo Community Association, Charlotte Despard Av,
Battersea, London SW11 5HD
Helpline: 0845 1200 660
email: office@famanon.org.uk
www.famanon.org.uk
Runs self-help groups in the UK and worldwide for families and friends of those
with a drug problem.

Narcotics Anonymous (worldwide)
UK Service Office, 202 City Rd, London EC1V 2PH
Office: Tel: 020 7251 4007
Fax: 020 7251 4006
email: ukso@ukna.org
Helpline: 020 7730 0009 (10am–10pm daily)
email: helpline@ukna.org
www.ukna.org
A network of recovering addicts supporting each other to live without drugs.

National Drugs Helpline/Talk to Frank
Helpline: 0800 776600 (24-hour)
Textphone: 0800 917 8765
email: frank@talktofrank.com
www.talktofrank.com
Provides free confidential drug information and advice, including information on local services.

National Treatment Agency for Substance Misuse
5th Floor, Hannibal House, Elephant and Castle, London
Telephone/Helpline: 020 7972 2214
email: nta.enquiries@nta.gsi.gov.uk
www.nta.nhs.uk
A special health authority established by the government to increase the availability, capacity and effectiveness of treatment for drug misuse in England. Offers advice and information.

Release
388 Old Street, London EC1V 9LT
Admin: Tel: 020 7729 5255
Fax: 020 2279 2599
Heroin and Legal Helpline: 0845 4500 215 (10am–5.30pm, Monday–Friday)
email: ask@release.org.uk
www.release.org.uk
Advice, support and information to drug users and their friends and families on all aspects of drug use and drug-related legal problems.

Eating disorders
National Centre for Eating Disorders (branches across the country)
54 New Rd, Esher, Surrey KT10 9NU
Tel: 01372 469493
www.eating-disorders.org.uk
Set up to provide solutions for all eating disorders. Counselling for individuals, information and training for professionals.

Eating Disorders Association (local groups)
103 Prince of Wales Road, Norwich NR1 1DW
Admin: Tel: 0870 770 3656

Fax: 0160 366 4951
email: info@edauk.com
Adult Helpline: 0845 634 1414 (8.30–18.30, Monday–Friday, 13.00–16.30 Saturday)
Adult email service: helpmail@edauk.com
Youthline (for under 18s): 0845 634 7650 (16.00–18.30, Monday–Friday, 13.00–16.30 Saturday)
Youth email service: talkback@ebauk.com
www.edauk.com
Self-help support groups for sufferers, their relatives and friends. Assists in putting people in touch with sources of help in their own area.

Gambling
Gamblers Anonymous
Main Telephone: 020 7384 3040
Southern Region: 020 7384 3040
Midlands Region: 0121 233 1335
North East Region: 01142 620 026
North West Region: 0161 976 5000
Scotland: 0141 630 1033
Ireland Derry: 01504 351 329
Dublin: 01 8721133
www.gamblersanonymous.org
This is an international fellowship of men and women who share their experience, strength and hope with each other that they may solve their common problem and help others to recover from a gambling problem. The only requirement for membership is a desire to stop gambling. Anonymous membership.

Parents and children
Contact a Family
209–211 City Road, London EC1V 1JN
Tel: 020 7608 8700
Fax: 020 7608 8701
Helpline: 0808 808 3555
Textphone: 0808 808 3556
(freephone for parents and families 10am–4pm Monday–Friday)
email: info@cafamily.co.uk
www.cafamily.co.uk
This charity provides support and advice to parents with disabled children, whatever the medical condition of the child.

NEWPIN (local groups, including NI)
National Newpin, Sutherland House, 35 Sutherland Sq, Walworth, London SE17 3EE
Tel: 020 7358 5900
Fax: 020 7701 2660

email: info@newpin.org.uk
www.newpin.org.uk
Works with families to help break the cycle of destructive behaviour. Befriending and support groups for parents of young children who are under stress. Work focuses on alleviating maternal depression and stress. Provides training in parenting skills and family play programmes.

Parentline Plus
Endway House, The Endway, Hadleigh, Essex SS7 2AN
Office: Tel: 01702 554 782
email: contact@parentlineplus.org.uk
Helpline: 0808 800 2222 (24 hours)
Textphone: 0800 783 6783 (9am–5pm, Monday–Friday)
www.parentlineplus.org.uk
Previously Parentline UK and The National Stepfamily Association, now merged into Parentline Plus. Offers help and advice to parents on all aspects of bringing up children and teenagers. Provides support for parents under stress.

Parents Anonymous (local groups)
36 Park Drive, London NW11 7SP
Tel: 020 7263 8918 (19.00–00.00 hours, most evenings)
Offers friendship and help to parents who are at risk of abusing their children and those who may have done so. Provides information, telephone counselling and visiting service for parents; network of local groups.

Young Minds
102–108 Clerkenwell Road, London EC1M 5SA
Tel: 020 7336 8445
Fax: 020 7336 8446
Parents Information service: Tel: 0800 018 2138
www.youngminds.org.uk
Produces books and leaflets about young people's mental health and offers seminars and training.

Personality disorders
Borderline UK
PO Box 42, Cockermouth, Cumbria CA13 0WB
email: info@borderlineuk.co.uk
www.borderlineuk.co.uk
A national user-led network of people within the UK who have been diagnosed with borderline personality disorder.

Borderline
www.bpdcentral.com
A list of resources for people who care about someone with borderline personality disorder.

Relationship problems
British Association for Sexual and Relationship Therapy (BASRT)
Tel/Fax: 020 8543 2707
email: info@basrt.org.uk
www.basrt.org.uk
Registered therapists are multidisciplinary and work in the NHS as well as privately.

Care for the Family
PO Box 488, Cardiff CF15 7YY
Tel: 029 2081 0800
Fax: 029 2081 4089
email: email@cff.org.uk
www.care-for-the-family.org.uk
Provides help for those experiencing distress from family problems.

The Sexual Dysfunction Association
Windmill Pl. Business Centre, 2–4 Windmill Lane, Southall, Middlesex UB2 4NJ
Helpline: 0870 774 3571
email: info@sda.uk.net
www.impotence.org.uk
Helps suffers of impotence and their partners.

Relate
Local branches across the UK including NI, the Isle of Man, Channel Islands and Scotland. Contact details for individual branches listed on website.
Helpline/Booking line: 08451 304 016 (8.30–4.30, Monday–Friday)
www.relate.org.uk
Relate offers advice, relationship counselling, sex therapy, workshops, meditation, support by face-to-face consultations, by phone and through information on the website.

Schizophrenia
Hearing Voices Groups (local groups)
email: bdhrg@hearingvoices.co.uk
www.hearingvoices.co.uk
Link to contacts for self-help groups to allow people to explore their voice-hearing experiences.

Rethink (formerly the National Schizophrenia Fellowship) (local groups)
28 Castle Street, Kingston-upon-Thames, Surrey KT1 1SS
General enquiries: Tel: 0845 456 0455
email: info@rethink.org
Advice line: 020 8974 6814 (10am–3pm, Monday–Friday)
email: advice@rethink.org
www.rethink.org
Works to help everyone affected by severe mental illness, including schizophrenia, to recover better quality of life. More than 300 services in England,

Wales and Northern Ireland provided, including home treatment, nursing care, carers' support, helplines and advocacy.

Schizophrenia Association of Great Britain
Bryn Hyfryd, The Crescent, Bangor, Gwynedd LL57 2AG
Tel: 01248 35 40 48
Fax: 01248 35 36 59
email: info@sagb.co.uk
www.sagb.co.uk
Offers information and support to sufferers, relatives, friends, carers and medical workers.

The UK NHS Portal for Schizophrenia
www.nelmh.org/home_schizophrenic.asp?c=10
Web-based information resource for people with schizophrenia and their carers. The site contains a number of user-friendly sections. These include the following: Evidence based treatment summaries; What is schizophrenia?; How is schizophrenia diagnosed?; Managing schizophrenia; Living with schizophrenia; Support for carers; and Legal issues.

Self-harm and suicide
Basement Project
PO Box 5, Abergavenny, Gwent NP7 5XW
Tel: 01873 856 524
email: basement.project@virgin.net
www.freespace.virgin.net/basement.project
Research into and publications about on self-harm, self-injury forum, training and workshops for professionals and work with people (mainly women) who have been abused.

Bristol Crisis Service for Women
PO Box 654, Bristol BS99 1XH
Admin: Tel: 0117 927 9600
Helpline: 0117 925 1119 (9pm–12.30am, Friday and Saturday)
email: bcsw@womens-crisis-service.freeserve.co.uk
Telephone counselling and information service relating to self-harm. Bi-monthly newsletter Shout on self-harm.

National Inquiry into Self-Harm among Young People
Camelot Foundation, University House, 13 Lower Grosvenor Place, London SW1W 0EX
Tel: 020 7828 6085
email: info@selfharmuk.org
www.selfharmuk.org
The national inquiry into self-harm is the UK's first major investigation into self-harm launched in March 2004 for 18 months. It aims to collate information into self-harm and can provide information on additional support for those who

self-harm, their family, friends and those who work with them. Any evidence about self-harm including personal experience is welcome.

National Self-Harm Network (NSHN)
PO Box 7264, Nottingham NG1 6WJ
email: info@nshn.co.uk
www.nshn.co.uk
Provides information sheets and training.

The Samaritans
46 Marshall Street, London W1F 9BF
Helpline: UK 08457 909090 and ROI 1850 60 9090 (24-hour, daily)
email: jo@samaritans.org
www.samaritans.org.uk
Offers confidential emotional support to any person who is despairing or suicidal. 203 local branches across the UK and ROI offer opportunity to talk face-to-face.

Self-Injury and Related Issues (SIARI)
email: jan@siari.uk
www.siari.co.uk
The website, owned by a counsellor, Jan Sutton, provides information on a wide range of topics relating to self-harm. Very useful and supportive information for suffers, families and professionals. Not a personal advice service.

SOBS (Survivors of Bereavement by Suicide) (local groups)
Centre 88, Saner Street, Hull HU3 2TR
Administrator: Tel: 01482 610 728
Fax: 01482 210287
email: sobsadmin@care4free.net
Helpline: 0870 241 3337 (9am–9pm, 365 days of the year)
email: sobs.support@care4free.net
www.uk-sobs.org.uk
Offers emotional and practical support to those affected by suicide.

Trauma
The Medical Foundation for the Care of Victims of Torture
111 Isledon Rd, Islington, London N7 7JW (open 9am–6pm, Monday–Friday, by appointment)
Tel: 020 7697 7777
Fax: 020 7697 7788
Clinical team email: clinical@torturecare.org.uk
www.torturecare.org.uk
Provides survivors of torture with medical treatment, social assistance and psychotherapeutic support.

Rape Crisis Federation
Tel: 0115 900 3560 (9am–5pm, Monday–Friday)
email: info@rapecrisis.co.uk
www.rapecrisis.co.uk

Victim Support and Witness Support
Cranmer House, 39 Brixton Rd, London SW9 6DZ
Office: Tel: 020 7735 9166
Fax: 020 7582 5712
email: contact@victimsupport.org.uk
Supportline: 0845 3030 900 (9am–9pm, Monday–Friday; 9am–7pm, Saturday/
Sunday; 9am–5pm bank holidays)
Support email: supportline@victimsupport.co.uk
www.victimsupport.com
Victim Support provides emotional support and practical information for anyone
who has suffered the effects of crime, regardless of whether the crime has been
reported. Witness Support provides support to witnesses of crime.

Women Against Rape (WAR) and Black Women's Rape Project (BWRAP)
Tel: 020 7482 2496
Fax: 020 7209 4761
email: war@womenagainstrape.net, bwrap@dircon.co.uk
www.womenagainstrape.net

Treatment: counselling and psychotherapy
The Association for Psychoanalytic Psychotherapy in the NHS
5 Windsor Road, London N3 3SN
Tel: 020 8349 9873
www.app-nhs.org.uk

British Association for Counselling and Psychotherapy (BACP)
BACP House, 35–37 Albert Street, Rugby, Warks CV21 2SG
Tel: 0870 443 5252
Fax: 0870 443 5161
www.counselling.co.uk
www.bacp.co.uk
Provides advice on sources of individual counselling and family therapy in the UK.

British Association for Behavioural and Cognitive Psychotherapies
Globe Centre, PO Box 9, Accrington BB5 2GD
Tel: 01254 875277
Fax: 01254 239114
email: babcp@babcp.com
www.babcp.org.uk
Provides a free directory of accredited cognitive behavioural practitioners.

British Association of Psychotherapies
37 Mapesbury Road, London
Tel: 020 8452 9823
Fax: 020 8452 5182
ermail: mail@bap-psychotherapy.org
www.bap-psychotherapy.org

The British Confederation of Psychotherapists
West Hill House, Swains Lane, London N6 6QS
Tel: 020 7267 3626
Fax: 020 7267 4772
email: mail@bcp.org.uk
www.bcp.org.uk
Register of psychotherapists, including psychoanalysts, analytical psychologists, psychoanalytical psychotherapists and child psychotherapists.

The British Psychological Society
St Andrew's House, 48 Princess Road East, Leicester LE1 7DR
Tel: 0116 254 9568
Fax: 0116 247 0787
email: enquiry@bps.org.uk
www.bps.org.uk
Produces a directory of chartered clinical psychologists.

Counsellors and Psychotherapists in Primary Care (CPC)
Queensway House, Queensway, Bognor Regis, West Sussex PO21 1QT
Tel: 01243 870701
Fax: 01243 870702
email: cpc@cpc-online.co.uk
www.cpc-online.co.uk
Represents counsellors and psychotherapists working in the NHS as a self-regulating professional association.

Institute for Counselling and Personal Development Trust
Interpoint, 20–24 York Street, Belfast BT15 1AQ
Tel: 02890 330 996
email: icpd@btconnect.com
Offers counselling and psychotherapy (normally free), a course for helpers and community training and development courses.

United Kingdom Council for Psychotherapy (UKCP)
167–169 Great Portland Street, London W1W 5PF
Tel: 020 7436 3002
Fax: 020 7436 3013
email: ukcp@psychotherapy.org.uk
www.psychotherapy.org.uk
Provides information on registered therapists and training organisations.

Complementary medicine

While many practising doctors are sceptical as to the usefulness of complementary medical interventions, the feedback from sick doctors who have experienced effects from such treatment is often very positive. It is important to choose a practitioner who is registered with and approved by the relevant professional body. The following list cannot be inclusive of all therapies available and only a selection of contacts is given.

The British Holistic Medical Association
59 Landsdown Place, Hove, East Sussex BN3 1FL
Tel: 01273 725951
email: bhma@bhma.org
www.bhma.org

The Institute for Complementary Medicine
PO Box 194, London SE16 1QZ
Tel: 020 7237 5165
Fax: 020 7237 5175
email: info@icmedicine.co.uk
www.icmedicine.co.uk

Acupuncture

British Medical Acupuncture Society (BMAS)
BMAS House, 3 Winnington Court, Northwich, Cheshire CW8 1AQ
(medically qualified acupuncturists)
Tel: 01606 786782
Fax: 01606 786783
email: Admin@medical-acupuncture.org.uk
www.medical-acupuncture.co.uk

British Acupuncture Council
63 Jeddo Road, London W12 9HQ
Tel: 020 8735 0400
Fax: 020 8735 0404
email: info@acupuncture.org.uk
www.acupuncture.org.uk

Aromatherapy

International Federation of Professional Aromatherapists (IFPA)
82 Asby Road, Hickley, Leicestershire LE10 1SN
Tel: 01455 637987
email: admin@IFPAroma.org
www.ifparoma.org

Homeopathy

The British Homeopathic Association, the Faculty of Homeopathy, Homeo-pathic Trust
Hahnemann House, 29 Park Street West, Luton LU1 3BE

Tel: 0870 444 3950
Fax: 0870 444 3960
www.trusthomeopathy.org
NHS Homeopathic Hospitals can be found in Bristol, Liverpool, Glasgow, London and Tunbridge Wells. For more information including how to refer via GP, contact as above.

The Homeopathic Medical Association
Administration Office, 6 Livingstone Road, Gravesend, Kent DA12 5DZ
Tel: 01474 560336
email: info@the-hma.org
www.the-hma.org

Hypnosis

The British Society of Medical and Dental Hypnosis
Tel: 07000 56039
www.bsmdh.org

Further reading

BBC health information: Mental Health pages
www.bbc.co.uk/health/mental
Provides useful advice on mental health and related health issues, including further resources and self-help advice.

NHS National electronic Library for Health
www.nel.nhs.co.uk

NHS National electronic Library for Mental Health
www.nelmh.org

National Institute for Mental Health in England (NIMHE)
www.nimhe.org.uk

Mental Health Care
www.mentalhealthcare.org.uk
Information about mental health and the latest research from the South London and Maudsley NHS Trust and the Institute of Psychiatry. Particularly suited to the carers, friends and family of anyone with mental illness. The site currently deals with schizophrenia and psychosis.

Patient UK
www.patient.co.uk
A directory of UK health, diseases, illness and related websites providing patient information and support.

Surgery Door
www.surgerydoor.co.uk
Comprehensive list of 200 support groups in the UK.

WHO Collaborating Centre for Mental Health Research and Training (2004)
WHO Guide to Mental Health and Neurological Health in Primary Care.
A guide to mental and neurological ill health in adults, adolescents and children.
Adapted for the UK from *Diagnostic and Management Guidelines for Mental Disorders in Primary Care*: ICD 10, Chapter V Primary Care Version.
WHO Collaborating Centre for Mental Health Research and Training, Institute of Psychiatry, King's College, The Royal College of Psychiatrists, The Royal College of General Practitioners, The Royal College of Physicians Joint Committee for Neurology, The Royal College of Nursing, NIMHE (National Institute for Mental Health in England), Neurological Alliance, European Federation of Neurological Associations, The Patients Association, PriMHE (Primary Care Mental Health Education), Mental Health Nurses Association, The Association of Counsellors and Psychotherapists in Primary Care, The Queen's Nursing Institute, Community Practitioners' and Health Visitors' Association.
The Royal Society of Medicine Press
ISBN 1-85315-560-8
www.mentalneurologicalprimarycare.org

References

1   AAGBI (1997) *Stress in the Anaesthetist.* AAGBI, London.
2   Redfern N and Harrison J (2001) Flexible Training Scheme for doctors with chronic ill health. *BMJ career focus.* **322**: 52–7296.
3   Mersey Deanery website: www.merseydeanery.ac.uk.
4   BMA Charities (2002) *Trustees' Report 1 January–31 December 2001.* BMA, London.
5   Chambers R, Schwartz E and Boath E (2002) *Beating Stress in the NHS.* Radcliffe Medical Press, Oxford.

Index

Ability on line 176
abuse 27, 28, 139, 179, 181
access to healthcare 52–3, 54, 137
Access to Work Scheme 162
accident and emergency medicine 121, 157
action plans for depression 108–9, 112
acupuncture 187
addictions
    Disability Discrimination Act 138
    GMC Health Procedures 91, 94
    personal accounts 5, 71
    resources 146, 155, 172, 177–8
ADFAM International 178
admission to hospital *see* hospitalisation
adolescents 45, 78, 170, 179, 182
affective disorders
    medical students 73
    personal accounts 5, 10, 33, 41, 85
    resources 106, 154
African Caribbean Mental Health
    Association (ACMHA) 169
alcohol 11, 15, 16, 92, 138, 155, 171–2
Allitt, Beverley 135
anaesthetists 154, 157
anorexia 27–8, 71 *see also* eating disorders
antidepressants
    personal accounts 9–12, 16, 33, 35, 86,
        88
    relapse prevention 106, 109
    stigma 65
anxiety
    personal accounts 3, 25, 26, 67, 86
    relapse prevention 112
    resources 170–1, 173
application forms 64–5, 77–8, 85, 147,
    165
aromatherapy 117, 187
art therapy 16, 17, 27, 28
Asian community resources 171, 176
Association for Postnatal Illness 176
Association for Psychoanalytic
    Psychotherapy in the NHS 185
Association of Anaesthetists of GB and
    Ireland (AAGBI) 154, 157
Association of Disabled Professionals 176
Association of Managers of Student
    Services in Higher Education
    (AMOSSHE) 77

asylum seekers 125, 128
Aware Defeat Depression 175

Balint, Michael 53
Basement Project 183
BBC health pages 188
benefits advice
    personal accounts 28–9, 85
    resources 128, 133, 146, 164–5, 175
benzodiazepines 32, 177
bereavement 4, 23–4, 182
bingeing 25, 26, 70, 71 *see also* bulimia
bipolar disorder 10, 91, 106, 138, 174
bizarre thinking 68–9, 108
black community resources 168, 185
BMA (British Medical Association)
    charities 133, 165
    counselling 54, 154
    Disability Discrimination Act 76, 138,
        143
    employment issues 138, 143, 160, 162
    GMC Health Procedures 93
    stigma and discrimination 64
BMJ (British Medical Journal) 33, 146, 155,
    162
borderline personality disorder 181–2 *see
    also* personality disorder
Bristol Crisis Service for Women 183
British Acupuncture Council 187
British Association for Behavioural and
    Cognitive Psychotherapies 185
British Association for Counselling and
    Psychotherapy (BACP) 185
British Association for Sexual and
    Relationship Therapy (BASRT) 182
British Association of Psychotherapies 185
British Doctors' and Dentists' Group 155
British Holistic Medical Association 187
British Homeopathic Association 187–8
British Medical Acupuncture Society
    (BMAS) 187
British Medical Association *see* BMA
British Medical Journal see BMJ
British Psychological Society 186
British Society of Medical and Dental
    Hypnosis 187
bulimia 25, 27, 71, 72, 101
burn-out xi, 7, 13, 31, 40

Cameron Fund 166
Campaign Against Living Miserably
  (CALM) 175
Care for the Family 182
career choice
  career planning 143–4
  medical students 79, 80, 82
  and mental illness 39–41, 63
  personal accounts 5, 7, 10–11, 15, 41–2,
    87
  relapse prevention 111
  resources 147, 156–63
carers' resources 174–5, 181
catastrophisation 67
C.A.U.S.E. for Mental Health 169
CBT *see* cognitive behaviour therapy
Changing Minds campaign 64
charities 28, 133, 164
childcare 34, 47, 126, 128, 129
children
  abuse 27
  childhood disorders 33, 78
  resources 158, 170, 171–2, 179, 184
Chronic Illness Matching Scheme 155
CITA (Council for Involuntary
    Tranquilliser Addiction) 178
Citizens Advice Bureau 166
Clothier Report 135, 137
cognitive behaviour therapy (CBT)
  career planning 144
  flexible working 125, 128
  personal accounts 16, 20, 28, 35, 68,
    86, 89
  relapse prevention 109
  resources 153, 184
cognitive distortions 67–9, 88
colleagues
  employment issues 128, 144
  human support 48–9, 53
  issues in treatment 51–3, 55
  medical schools and students 79, 81
  relapse prevention 110–11
  talking to 43, 70, 87
  trust 68–9
Community Psychiatric Nurses (CPNs) 19,
    71, 109, 112, 120, 128
Community Safety Unit 176
compensation 76, 166
complaints procedures 34, 46
complementary medicine 186–8
conduct procedures (GMC) 45, 64, 91, 92,
    94, 147
confidentiality

GMC Health Procedures 92, 93, 94
  medical schools and students 75, 77, 79,
    80, 82
  Occupational Health 142, 143
  personal accounts 36, 44–5, 88
  resources 147, 152–5
  stigma 51–2, 64
Contact a Family 180
contingency plans 34, 52, 128
continuity of care 43–5, 52
co-ops 123, 131, 134
coping with mental illness
  being 'selfish'? 119–20
  keeping it contained 116–17
  keeping it simple 115–16
  self-harm 122
  suicidal thoughts 120–2
  use of symbolism/imagination 117–19
  use of the senses 117
Council for Involuntary Tranquilliser
    Addiction (CITA) 177
counselling
  medical schools and students 74, 79
  personal accounts 28, 33, 35, 54, 62, 71
  resources 152–4, 170, 171, 176, 186–7
Counsellors and Psychotherapists in
    Primary Care (CPC) 186
countertransference 89
course organisers 55, 127, 128
Cox, Heidi 75
CPNs *see* Community Psychiatric Nurses
critical illness cover 123, 132
Crossroads Assocation 175
culture of medicine
  Doctors' Support Network 146–8
  DOH guidelines 137
  medical schools and students 73, 80, 82
  partnerships 123–4, 127–9
  prevalence of mental illness 4, 7
  stigma and discrimination 61–3, 65
  teamwork 53–4
cutting (self-harm) 70, 71, 72, 122

Dain Fund 165
Data Protection Act 1998 75
DDA *see* Disability Discrimination Act
deaneries
  careers advice 143, 156, 160, 161
  flexible working 48, 126, 127
  medical schools and students 82
  recruitment 54–5
  resources 152–3, 156, 160, 161, 167
debt resources 174

deeds of partnership 62–3, 123–4
defence organisations 93, 166
dentists 153, 155, 167, 186
Department for Work and Pensions
     (DWP) 162, 166, 167
Department of Health (DOH)
   employment issues xi, 56, 136–7, 142–3
   GMC Health Procedures 92
   resources 155, 161
   stigma and discrimination 64
depersonalisation 32
depression *see also* coping with mental
     illness
   Doctors' Support Network 146, 148
   easily misunderstood experiences 67,
     68, 71
   employment issues 26, 127, 144
   financial costs of illness 131, 134
   personal accounts 9–13, 15–16, 19–22,
     31–6, 53, 85–9
   prevalence in doctors 3–5, 7
   relapse prevention 106–9, 112
   resources 170, 175–6, 179
de-realisation 33–5, 68
diaries 71, 118
diet 9, 10, 71, 116, 117, 122 *see also* eating
     disorders
disability *see also* Disability Discrimination
     Act
   employment issues 136, 137–40, 141,
     143
   medical schools and students 73–4,
     76–83
   prevalence of mental illness 4
   resources 155, 162, 166, 176
Disability Conciliation Service 76
Disability Discrimination Act 1995 (DDA)
     see also disability
   Doctors' Support Network 146, 147
   employment issues 136, 137–40, 142,
     143
   medical schools and students 73–6
   resources 152, 162
   stigma and discrimination 63, 65
Disability Rights Commission (DRC) 76,
     83, 143, 163, 176
DisabledGo 177
disclosure of disability 75–6, 78–81, 88,
     138, 147
disconnections 67–9
discrimination *see also* Disability
     Discrimination Act
   Doctors' Support Network 148

employment issues 136–9, 141
   medical schools and students 73–7, 81–3
   and stigma 61–6
diurnal variation 106, 108, 111
DIVERSE project 82
Doctor Patient Partnership (DPP) 168
doctor patients *see also* doctors
   employment issues 135
   personal accounts 12, 25–9, 37–8, 85–9,
     98
   resources 152
   stigma and discrimination 64, 65
   treatment 55–6
doctors *see also* doctor patients
   coping with mental illness 118, 120
   depression 11–12, 19, 21–2, 24
   employment issues 41–2, 47–8, 54–5
   financial costs of illness 131, 132, 133
   GMC referral 24, 91–3
   health service problems 42–6
   issues in treatment 51–7
   mentoring 80
   need for own GP 43, 54, 111–12, 120,
     151
   need for support 48–9
   prevalence of mental illness 3–5, 7, 11,
     73, 77–8
   relapse prevention 111–12
   resources 151, 152–4
   self-treatment 42
   shame and vulnerability 41
   stigma and discrimination 63
Doctors in Difficulties (Mersey Deanery)
     156
Doctors' Support Line (DSL) 65, 121, 146,
     148, 149, 155
Doctors' Support Network (DSN)
   contact details 149
   employment issues 40, 136
   GMC Health Procedures 93
   history and background xi, 145–9
   personal accounts 21, 54
   relapse prevention 109, 111
   resources 115, 154–5
   stigma and discrimination 63, 64, 65
DOH *see* Department of Health
domestic violence 177–8
Down Your Drink 172
drama therapy 27
DRC *see* Disability Rights Commission
Drinkline National Alcohol Helpline 172
drug misuse 73, 138, 143, 178–9 *see also*
     self-prescribing

DSL *see* Doctors' Support Line
DSMIV (Diagnostic and Statistical Manual of Mental Disorders, Fourth Edition) 62
DSN *see* Doctors' Support Network
DWP *see* Department for Work and Pensions

eating disorders
    de-realisation 68
    personal accounts 9–10, 21, 25–8, 32, 41, 100–1
    prevalence in doctors 5, 73
    relapse prevention 106, 117
    resources 179–80
    self-harm 70–2, 122
ECT (electroconvulsive therapy) 15, 19, 21, 36
email forums 121, 146, 147–8, 154
emergencies 52, 121, 157
empathy 7, 70, 86, 89, 111, 118
employment issues
    beyond the Clothier Report 135–6
    career planning 143–4
    Disability Discrimination Act 137–40
    Doctors' Support Network 147
    DOH guidelines for NHS 136–7
    flexible working 140–1
    GMC Health Procedures 93
    human rights 141
    Occupational Health Services 141–3, 151–2
    students' transition to work 82
Employment Medical Advisory Service (EMAS) 164
Emson, Daksha 82, 135, 136
Everyman Project 177
examinations (academic) 4, 25–6, 31, 35, 74–5, 164
exercise 10, 128

Faculty of Family Planning and Reproductive Healthcare 158
Faculty of Occupational Medicine of the Royal College of Physicians 94, 152, 158
Faculty of Public Health Medicine 159
failure, feeling a 5, 10, 16, 93
faith 17, 27, 111, 119
family
    career planning 144
    medical schools and students 79, 80
    prevalence of mental illness 5, 11

relapse prevention 110, 111, 112
    resources 158, 178, 179, 183
    stigma and confidentiality 51
    support networks 48–9, 121
financial issues 26, 85, 131–4, 140, 146, 165–7
First Steps to Freedom 173
'fitness to enter' schemes 77–8, 82
fitness to practise
    GMC Health Procedures 91, 92, 93
    medical schools and students 73, 81–2
    and mental illness 39–41
    Occupational Health Services 142, 143
    relapse prevention 109–10, 111
    resources 159
Flexible Careers Scheme 28–9, 124, 126, 129, 140, 160–1 *see also* flexible working
flexible training 26, 48, 63, 126, 156, 161
flexible working *see also* Flexible Careers Scheme
    deaneries 126
    Doctors' Support Network 147
    mental health and employment 139–41, 143
    partnerships 123–5
    personal accounts 10, 34, 47–8, 56
    The Project Surgery 127–9
    resources 126–7
    salaried practitioners 125–6
    stigma and discrimination 63, 65
fluoxetine (Prozac) 19, 71
food 9, 10, 71, 116, 117, 122 *see also* eating disorders
Food and You 122
foreign doctors' resources 166–7
freelance GPs 123, 131, 132, 134
friends (support networks) 48–9, 51, 70, 79–80, 110–13, 121, 144

gambling 180
Gay and Lesbian Association of Doctors and Dentists (GLADD) 168
General Medical Council (GMC)
    Doctors' Support Network 147
    Health Procedures 91–4
    medical schools and students 75, 81
    personal accounts 23–4, 26, 45
    resources 151, 159–60, 164
    stigma and discrimination 64, 65
general practice 7, 13, 54, 55, 126, 157
Gestalt therapy 27

GMC *see* General Medical Council
GPs (general practitioners) *see* doctor
    patients; doctors
guilt 25, 31, 93
gynaecology resources 158

hallucinations 32, 34
hanging (suicide) 12, 71
harassment 139, 163
Hastings Benevolent Fund 164
Health and Safety 142, 151–2, 164–5
Health Development Agency (HDA) 163
Health Procedures (GMC) 91–4, 159–60
health resources 65, 167–8
health screening 24, 45, 54, 91–3, 135,
    137
Healthy Return to Work 162–3
Healthy Workplaces 136
Hearing Voices Groups 182
homeopathy 187–8
homosexual doctors' resources 168
hospitalisation
    employment issues 40
    financial costs of illness 134
    medical schools and students 77–8
    misunderstood experiences 69, 71
    personal accounts 12, 15, 19, 21, 27–8,
        33, 35
    prevalence of mental illness 3
    relapse prevention 112
    stigma and confidentiality 51–2
    treating doctor patients 27–8, 37–8, 56,
        87
House Concern 152–3
housing advice 166
human rights 77, 136, 141
hypnosis 188

ICD-10 (International Classification of
    Diseases, Tenth Revision) 62
identity 106–7, 147
imagery 16, 117–19, 121
Improving Working Lives 140, 147
income
    financial costs of illness 28–9, 131–4
    insurance 123, 132, 134
    resources 156, 164–6
Injury Benefit Scheme 133, 134
insight 53, 65, 68–9, 111, 143
Institute for Complementary Medicine
    185
Institute for Counselling and Personal
    Development Trust 186

Institute of Psychiatry 187
insurance
    Disability Discrimination Act 140
    financial costs of illness 131, 132, 134
    flexible working 123, 125
    GMC Health Procedures 94
    resources 111, 164
    sectioning 89
    stigma and discrimination 61
Intensive Care Society 157
International Doctors in Alcoholics
    Anonymous (IDAA) 155
International Federation of Professional
    Aromatherapists (IFPA) 187
International Stress Management
    Association (ISMA) 164, 173

Jobcentre Plus 29, 162
jobsharing 141, 161–2
Joint Committee on Postgraduate Training
    and General Practice 157
junior doctors 4, 26, 56, 64, 80, 82

Kiran: Asian Women's Aid 177

learning disabilities 29, 168
legal resources 164–6, 178
lesbian doctors' resources 167
lists 116–17, 121
lithium 21, 43, 86, 99, 128
locums
    financial costs of illness 131, 132, 134
    flexible working 47, 128
    GMC Health Procedures 92
    personal accounts 13, 34, 47, 56
    resources 160
    stigma and discrimination 61
London Lighthouse 79

Manic Depression Fellowship (MDF) 174
manic episodes 69, 86, 107–8, 138, 140
mantras 119
Maudsley Hospital 52, 154, 187
MDF (Manic Depression Fellowship) 174
MDU (Medical Defence Union) 167
Medical Benevolent Fund 133, 146, 164
Medical Council on Alcoholism 155, 172
medical defence organisations 93, 166
Medical Forum 143, 160
Medical Foundation for the Care of
    Victims of Torture 184
Medical Protection Society (MPS) 23, 24
medical schools
    applications and admissions 64, 77–8

medical schools (*cont.*)
  and disability 73–6, 78–9
  fitness to practise 81–2
  legislation 76–7
  seeking help 79–81
  transition to work 82–3
Medical Women's Federation 168
medication *see also* self-prescribing
  Disability Discrimination Act 138
  GMC referral 24, 92
  personal accounts 10, 16, 19, 33, 52, 86
  relapse prevention 109, 111
  resources 151
MedNet 55, 153
membership fees 29, 156
memory 116, 118, 121, 138
Mental Health Act 1983 (MHA) 19, 62,
  85, 87, 89, 124, 141
Mental Health Care 188
Mental Health Foundation 169
mental illness *see also* coping with mental
  illness
  beyond the Clothier Report 135–6
  career planning 143–4
  Disability Discrimination Act 137–40
  doctor patients 55–6, 85–9
  DOH guidelines for NHS 136–7
  employment issues 39–42
  financial costs of illness 131–4
  flexible working 47–8, 140–1
  health service problems 42–5
  issues in treatment 51–7
  misunderstood experiences 67–72
  Occupational Health Services 141–3
  prevalence in doctors 3–5, 7, 11, 73,
    77–8
  resources 168–70
  stigma and discrimination 51–3, 61–6
  support networks 48–9
mentoring 55, 80, 82, 160
MHA *see* Mental Health Act
Michelson, Dr Soames 146
MIND 21, 169
mortgages 127, 131, 132
mother and baby units 21, 22, 45
MPs (members of parliament) 166
MPS (Medical Protection Society) 23, 24
music 17, 26, 29, 117, 119

Narcotics Anonymous 179
National Assembly for Wales 92
National Association for Children of
  Alcoholics (NACOA) 172

National Carers Association 173–4
National Centre for Eating Disorders 179
National Counselling Service for Sick
  Doctors 35, 153
National Debtline 175
National Domestic Violence Help Line 176
National Drugs Helpline/Talk to Frank 179
National Electronic Library for (Mental)
  Health 186
National Health Pension Agency 166
National Health Service *see* NHS
National Inquiry into Self-Harm among
  Young People 183–4
National Institute for Mental Health in
  England (NIMHE) 188
National Schizophrenia Fellowship 169,
  181
National Self-Harm Network (NSHN) 184
National Stepfamily Association 179
National Treatment Agency for Substance
  Misuse 179
National Union of Students (NUS) 76, 79
New Deal for Communities (NDC) 127
NEWPIN 180–1
NHS (National Health Service)
  Doctors' Support Network 147
  employment issues 135–7, 142, 144
  financial costs of illness 131
  GMC Health Procedures 94
  health service problems 42–6
  medical schools and students 78, 82–3
  pension scheme 131–4, 165
  prevalence of mental illness 4
  resources 153, 163, 185, 186, 188
NHS Professionals 140, 160, 161, 167
No Panic 173
North Ireland Community Addiction
  Service 172–3
Northern Ireland Association for Mental
  Health (NIAMH) 170
notebooks 116, 118
NUS (National Union of Students) 76, 79

obsessive-compulsive disorder 112, 172–3
obstetrics resources 158
Occupational Health Services
  Doctors' Support Network 146, 147
  GMC Health Procedures 94
  medical schools and students 77, 78, 82
  mental health and employment 135–7,
    141–3
  personal accounts 31, 36, 41, 44, 54
  prevalence of mental illness 5, 7

resources 151–2, 158, 161–3
  stigma and discrimination 64, 65
OCD Action 173
on-call work 97, 131, 134, 161
ophthalmology resources 158
out-of-hours (OOH) care 123, 126, 131, 134
overdoses 12, 19, 21, 33, 69–70, 88 *see also* suicide
overeating 25, 26, 28, 122 *see also* bingeing; bulimia
overseas doctors 166–7

paediatrics 158
panic disorders 117, 119, 138, 172–3
paranoia 34, 68, 108
parenting issues 5, 52–3, 136, 141, 181
paroxetine 33, 52
partnerships
  deeds 62–3, 123–4
  employment issues 39, 41
  financial costs of illness 131
  flexible working 123–5, 127–9
  prevalence of mental illness 4
  stigma and discrimination 61–3
  trust 68–9
part-time work 124, 126, 140, 156, 161–3
pathology resources 158
Patient UK 188
patients *see also* doctor patients
  emotional distance from 118–19
  health service problems 42–5
  resources 167–8
  safety 13, 24, 94, 136, 139, 142
  stigma and discrimination 64
PCTs (primary care trusts) 52, 126, 127, 148
pensions 131–4, 162, 165, 166
performance procedures (GMC) 91, 94, 147, 160
personalisation 68, 88
personality disorder (PD) 34, 62, 68, 87, 112, 135, 180
personality testing 78, 143
phobias 172–3
physiotherapy 140
plans (coping with depression) 107–9, 111, 112, 121, 122
postgraduate training 82, 140, 156, 162
postnatal depression 21, 55, 175, 179
pregnancy 9–10, 21, 22, 127
prejudice
  Doctors' Support Network 147
  employment issues 136, 144
  medical schools and students 78, 81

personal accounts 32, 56
prevalence of mental illness 4
self-harm 72
stigma and discrimination 61–3, 65
premises 125, 137, 140
prevalence of mental illness 3–5, 7, 11, 73, 77–8
primary care 43, 44, 82, 89, 127, 184
primary care trusts *see* PCTs
PriMHE (Primary Care Mental Health Education) 146, 155
private healthcare 44, 46, 78, 82
The Project Surgery 124, 127
Prozac (fluoxetine) 19, 71
psychiatric treatment
  employment issues 40, 82, 143
  GMC referral 23, 91, 93
  personal accounts 9–10, 12, 15–16, 19, 23, 27
  relapse prevention 109, 112, 120
  resources 159
  stigma and discrimination 64
psychoanalysis 55, 140, 183, 184
psychologists 10, 20, 143, 144, 184
psychometric testing 23, 36, 78, 160
psychotherapy
  flexible working 128
  personal accounts 24, 26, 34, 87
  prevalence of mental illness 4, 7
  resources 152–4, 183–5
  self-harm 71
psychotic illness 35, 40, 68, 86, 108, 187
public health medicine 27–9, 159
purging 25, 70

radiology resources 159
rape 28, 184–5
reality checking 69, 107
recruitment of staff 41, 54–5, 129
recurrent affective disorder 106
recurrent depression
  employment issues 40, 126, 128, 138
  personal accounts 9, 10, 20, 86
  relapse prevention 106, 108–9, 111
Red Book system 125, 131
Red Cross 122
Refuge 177
Refugee Doctor Liaison Group 167
relapse prevention
  depending on others 111–13
  early warning signs 110–11
  knowing oneself and the illness 107–10
  overview 105–7

Relate 177, 182
relationships 15–16, 68–9, 112, 170,
    176–7, 180
relaxation 115, 119
Release 179
religion 17, 27, 111, 119
reproductive healthcare 158
research 28, 29, 63, 64, 125
resources
    alcohol 170–2
    anxiety, OCD, panic and phobias 172–3
    bipolar disorder 173
    careers advice 156–63
    carers 173–4
    complementary medicine 185–6
    counselling and psychotherapy 183–5
    depression 174–5
    disability issues 175–6
    doctors from overseas 166–7
    doctors' professional services 152–4
    domestic violence 176–7
    drug misuse 177–8
    eating disorders 178–9
    financial and legal issues 164–6, 174
    further reading 186–7
    general health 151–2, 167–8
    general mental health 168–70
    Health and Safety at Work 163–4
    homosexual doctors 167
    Occupational Health Services 151–2
    parents and children 179
    personality disorders 180
    relationship problems 180
    schizophrenia 180–1
    self-harm and suicide 181–2
    self-help and peer support 154–5
    trauma 183
    women doctors 167
retention of staff 19, 41, 48, 65, 126, 129
Rethink 170, 182–3
retirement 13, 62, 131, 161, 164
returning to work
    Doctors' Support Network 147
    employment issues 140, 142, 144
    financial costs of illness 132, 133–4
    flexible working 47, 126
    personal accounts 20, 28, 33, 36, 56
    resources 152, 161, 162–3
    stigma and discrimination 64
revalidation 64, 65, 140, 160
rights
    disability 76, 83, 138, 143
    employment issues 136, 138, 141

human rights 77, 136, 141
    medical schools and students 76, 77, 79,
        83
    and safety 94, 163
risk to patients/self 13, 82, 88–9, 94, 142,
    143
Royal Colleges 64, 80, 94, 147, 152,
    156–9
Royal Medical Benevolent Fund 133, 146,
    165
Royal Society of Medicine 158
Rural Minds 169

SAD (Seasonal Affective Disorder)
    Association 176
salaried practitioners 48, 125–6, 131
The Samaritans 121, 184
SANE 170
scarring (self-harm) 70, 71, 72, 122
schizophrenia 138, 169, 182–3, 187
Scottish Association for Mental Health 170
screening see health screening
Seasonal Affective Disorder (SAD)
    Association 175
secondary care 43–4, 54, 82, 89, 111–12
sectioning (MHA) 19, 62, 71, 87–9, 124
self-employed GPs 123, 131, 132, 134
self-esteem
    coping with mental illness 116
    Doctors' Support Network 147
    issues in treatment 51
    personal accounts 9–10, 15, 25, 27–8,
        39, 42
self-harm
    coping with mental illness 119, 122
    misunderstood experiences 68, 69–72
    personal accounts 34
    relapse prevention 108, 110
    resources 183–4
self-help resources 154–5, 172
Self-Injury and Related Issues (SIARI) 184
self-prescribing 33, 42, 52–3, 151
self-referral 3, 35, 94, 142, 152–4
SENDA (Special Educational Needs and
    Disability Act) 2001 73
senses, use of 117, 118
sexual abuse 27, 28, 139
sexual therapy 176, 182
shame
    GMC Health Procedures 93
    personal accounts 11, 25, 39, 41–5
    self-harm 70, 72
    stigma and discrimination 65

Shelter 167
Sick Doctors' Trust 146, 154, 155
sickness absence
   Doctors' Support Network 147
   employment issues 135, 142–3
   financial costs of illness 131–4, 164
   personal accounts 21, 25, 35
   relapse prevention 109
   stigma and discrimination 62
Skill 74, 75, 76, 82
sleep problems 31–2, 53, 88, 108
SOBS (Survivors of Bereavement by
   Suicide) 184
Social Anxiety UK 173
social services 166–7
Someone To Talk To 170–1
Special Educational Needs and Disability
   Act 2001 (SENDA) 73
Spence, Christopher 79
spirituality 17, 27, 111, 119
SSRIs (selective serontonin reuptake
   inhibitors) 21, 35
stigma
   and access 52–3
   and confidentiality 51–2
   and discrimination 61–6
   Doctors' Support Network 146, 147
   employment issues 135, 136
   medical schools and students 73, 77, 78,
     80, 82
   personal accounts 26, 32, 39, 42, 45, 86
   prevalence of mental illness xi–xii, 4–5
   relapse prevention 109
   resources 154
stress
   employment issues 40, 128, 144
   medical schools and students 82
   personal accounts 10, 13, 25, 31, 54, 87
   prevalence of mental illness 3, 4, 5
   resources 116, 160, 164, 170, 173–4
   stigma and discrimination 53, 63
students
   applications and admissions 64, 77–8
   Disability Discrimination Act 73–6
   disclosure 78–9
   fitness to practise 81–2
   legislation 76–7
   resources 155, 165
   seeking help 79–81
   transition to work 82–3
substance misuse 73, 138, 143, 177–8
suicide
   coping with mental illness 120–2

financial costs of illness 134
GMC Health Procedures 91
mental health and employment 135
misunderstood experiences 69, 71
personal accounts 9, 12, 19, 21, 40–1,
   86–8
prevalence of mental illness 3–5
relapse prevention 106–8
resources 181–2
superannuation *see* pensions
supervision
   employment issues 129, 140, 161
   GMC referral 24, 92, 93
   personal accounts 7, 16, 21, 24
   stigma and discrimination 62, 64
support
   coping with mental illness 117–18, 121,
     122
   depending on others 111–13
   Doctors' Support Network 145–9
   employment issues 47–8, 128
   GMC Health Procedures 93
   knowing oneself and the illness 107–10
   medical schools and students 74, 77,
     79–80, 82
   need for own GP 111–12
   new identity 106–7
   personal accounts 34, 47–9, 53
   picking up early warning signs 110–11
   prevalence of mental illness 4–5
   resources 152–5, 187
   stigma and discrimination 51, 53, 64
Surgery Door 189
surgery resources 159, 167
Survivors of Bereavement by Suicide
   (SOBS) 184
symbolism 117–19, 121

Take Time 153
Talk to Frank/National Drugs Helpline 178
Tavistock Clinic 34, 153
torture 183
training *see also* medical schools; students
   disability 139–40
   Doctors' Support Network 147, 148
   employment issues 135, 139–40
   flexible training 26, 48, 63, 126, 156,
     161
   flexible working 48, 126, 127, 129
   personal accounts 9, 13, 21, 54–5
   prevalence of mental illness 4
   resources 151, 156, 160, 161
   stigma and discrimination 63

tranquillisers 177
transferences 87, 89, 113
trauma resources 184–5
treatment
  deanery recruitment 54–5
  doctor patients 37, 55–6
  in own hospital 36–7, 44–5, 51–2
  resources 185–6
  stigma 44–5, 51–3
  support 53–4
trichotillomania 172
Triumph over Phobia (TOP UK) 174
trust 68–9, 76, 128
tutors 55, 76, 79–80, 127, 144

UCAS forms 77, 78
unemployment 26, 28–9
unipolar affective disorder 33
United Kingdom Council for
    Psychotherapy (UKCP) 186
universities 75–7, 79–82, 125, 137

Victim Support 185
violence 143, 163, 176–7
vocational training schemes (VTS) 39, 55,
    87, 127
vomiting 25, 38, 70, 71, 72

warning signs of relapse 107–11

weight loss/gain 10–11, 25, 28, 32, 86
Witness Support 185
women's resources 168, 177–8, 185
Worker Webpage 164
working hours
  Disability Discrimination Act 139
  flexible working 47–8, 128, 141, 161
  medical schools and students 82
  personal accounts 26, 31
  prevalence of mental illness 4
  stigma and discrimination 63, 65
working parents 136, 141
working patterns *see also* flexible
    working
  career planning 143
  drive to work too hard 41–2
  flexible working 47–8
  medical schools and students 82–3
  personal accounts 10, 12–13, 16, 34,
    88–9
  resources 152, 161
  work–life balance 47, 136
work-related resources 156–63
Worst Kept Secret 178

young people's resources 45, 78, 170, 181,
    183–4

Zero Tolerance Campaign 164